USING GROUPWORK

Mark Doel

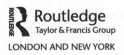
Routledge
Taylor & Francis Group
LONDON AND NEW YORK

communitycare

First published 2006
by Routledge
2 Park Square, Milton Park, Abingdon, Oxon, OX14 4RN

Simultaneously published in the USA and Canada
by Routledge
270 Madison Ave, New York NY 10016

Routledge is an imprint of the Taylor & Francis Group

Transferred to Digital Printing 2010

© 2006 Mark Doel

Typeset in Sabon and Futura
HWA Text and Data Management, Tunbridge Wells

British Library Cataloguing in Publication Data
A catalogue record for this book is available from the British Library

Library of Congress Cataloging in Publication Data
Doel, Mark.
Using groupwork / Mark Doel.
p.   cm.
Includes bibliographical references and index.
1. Social group work. 2. Group counselling. 3. Group relations
training. I. Title.
HV45.D65 2005
361.4–dc22
2005014295

ISBN10: 0–415–33931–6 (hbk)
ISBN10: 0–415–33932–4 (pbk)

ISBN13: 9–78–0–415–33931–5 (hbk)
ISBN13: 9–78–0–415–33932–2 (pbk)

This book is dedicated to my family group
for all their love, strength and playfulness

CONTENTS

BOXES

ACTIVITIES

ACKNOWLEDGEMENTS

This book would not have been possible without Catherine Sawdon, my colleague and co-tutor with the Groupwork Project. Catherine's support, enthusiasm and commitment to groupwork in particular and continuing professional development in general have been and continue to be inspiring. I would also like to thank Janet Atkinson, External Assessor for the Skills in Groupwork programme. Janet was a splendid critical friend to groupwork.

My thanks to all of the following people, mainly groupworkers in the project, for their participation and help, and all the learning that I derived from their experiences:

Jane Atwood, Carole Barlow, Caroline Barras, Paul Batty, Marion Beck, Sue Beedle, Wendy Bilinski, Susan Billingham, Julie Billington, Keith Birkhead, Barbara Bloomfield, Becky Broadbent, Helen Bromley, Georgia Cassar, Marie Castle, Steve Clow, Teresa Colley, Carol Cooper, Janet Cowley, Katherine Crawshaw, Maureen Dwyer, Lisa Evans, Simon Fagg, Sally Fawcett, Kim Finnerty, Lynne Flavell, Guy Fleming, Teresa Flood, Shirley Fothergill, Karen France, Ame Fu, Lorraine Garlick, Dilani Gaunt, Simon Gelder, Gail Gibbons, Jane Hardwick, Carol Harrison, Wendy Higgins, Peter Hirst, Maureen Horsfield, Marie Howells, Simon Hughes, Joanne Hutchinson, Diane Jewitt, Liz Jewitt, Helen Jillings, Lorraine Joy, Karen Kemp, Maria Kent, Wendy Kitchen, Jane Laycock, Sue Littledyke, Jackie Lonsdale, Michelle Loosemoor, Tim Lovell, Janet Mackintosh, Greg Maguire, Geraldine Marsh, Steve McAvoy, Denise McCulley, Cheryl McDougall, Donald McGovern, Tina McGuire, Bridie McHugh, Grazyna Melody, Katie Merrett, Lorna Miller, Gina Milne, Paul Milnes, Eamonn Mohans, Mark Monkman, Sue Moorehouse, Diane Morrison, Rachel Nelson, Mike Oldham, Vicki Ormondroyd, Keith Padgett, Shirley Palmer-Hunt, Janice Parker, Jackie Parnaby, Ann Pickard, Win Pidgeon, Ruth Queen, Steven Reed, Bernie Riordan, Damian Rules, Sara Rushworth, Lynne Ryan, John Ryden, Linda Sanderson, Jacqui Shuman, Sandra Siddall, Claire Sidebottom, Pete Simpson, Caroline Smith, Charlotte Smith (Hill), Duncan Smith, Sue Smithson, Darron Stone, Pat Stubbs, Janet Taylor, Sharon Terry, Anna Thomas, Julie Thompson, Melanie Thompson, Anne Thorpe, David Tulley, Julie Turner, Shaun Viney, Angela Wall (Ryton), Caroline Ward, Chrystal Ward, Jeremy Watson-Hunt, Pauline Watts, Julie Webb, Teresa Webb, Jayne Whittaker-Dakin, Christine Whittle, Lynn Wigham, Pauline Williams, Gillian Wilson, Maureen Wood and Janice Wootton.

CHAPTER 1

INTRODUCE

OBJECTIVES

By the end of this chapter you should:

▓ Feel introduced to the purpose, scope and limits of this book

▓ Know about the Groupwork Project and how it has informed this book

▓ Understand the nature of the portfolios used in this book

▓ Feel introduced to the groups which illustrate the book

▓ Be interested in the possibilities (and the limitations) of theorising from practice.

INTRODUCING THE BOOK

This book is about groupwork. It explores the similarities and differences between groups. Through that exploration the book seeks to develop an understanding of the nature of the 'groupwork' which unites these diverse experiences. As we shall see, the book makes regular and consistent reference to nine actual groups in order to learn more about the practice of groupwork. Through the lens of the groupworkers, we will learn more about the strengths and limitations of groups and about the many factors which contribute to a successful group.

Of equal importance to the groupworker's perspectives are those which derive from group members themselves and from formal research knowledge about groups and groupwork (Manor, 2000b). These perspectives will be incorporated into the text, though our principle viewpoint will be that of the groupworker, for reasons which will soon become clear.

I will be developing a model of groupwork which is 'generalist'. By this, I mean that it is not specific to any one kind of group in any one particular setting. It transfers readily to a broad variety of locations for groups and groupwork. The evidence for this claim comes from the experience of developing and refining the model of groupwork over many years with groups and groupworkers whose circumstances varied enormously. The contention that there are essential qualities common to all groupwork is based, therefore, on systematic experience and testing. Details of the Groupwork Project are contained in Box 1.1.

BOX   1.1   THE   GROUPWORK   PROJECT

The Groupwork Project was an action research project with the aim of developing and sustaining a groupwork service in a social work agency in northern England. The project was open to all staff in the agency, social workers and social care staff, and occasionally other professionals, in all sections and settings. It included a training and consultation programme over a period of half a year and this was integrated into a programme of continuing professional development. All participants were invited to submit portfolios of their groupwork practice for assessment. As noted, the quotations in this book are taken directly from a sample of nine of these portfolios. It is not the purpose of this book to present or evaluate the project as a whole, since this has been documented elsewhere (see below). Suffice it to say that, though the project had much success in generating groups and developing groupwork competence, when attempting to infiltrate the mainstream it encountered the kinds of difficulty which have been well documented by Smale (1996).

Further reading about the Groupwork Project:

Doel and Sawdon (1995, 1999a, 1999b); Doel et al. (2002).

The groups

68 groups were planned
54 groups ran successfully *(79% of those planned)*

Of the **54 groups** which ran successfully:
    37 groups were in community settings   *(69%)*
     9 groups were in day-care settings   *(17%)*
     7 groups were in residential settings   *(13%)*
     1 group was in a school setting   *(2%)*

    20 *(37%)* groups were in the children and families sector of which:
         1 *(+2)** groups with children below 12 yrs
        10 *(+1)** groups with young people 13–18 yrs

Box1.1 continued

      9 groups with carers of children and young people

      0 (+2)* groups with children with learning disabilities.

  14 (26%) groups were in the mental health sector; they included well-being, and not necessarily for people with diagnosed mental disorders.

    9 (17%) groups were in staff development.

    8 (15%) groups were in the adult services sector of which:

          7(+4)* groups with older people

          1(+1)* groups with adults with disabilities.

    3 (6%) groups were with offenders:

          1 group with adult offenders

          2 (+1)* groups with young offenders.

Figures in brackets indicated a related interest: for example, a group for parents and carers of young offenders is counted in the 'carers' tally and registered in brackets in the 'young offenders' category.

Percentages are rounded to the nearest whole number

Co-working

  47 groups had co-workers   *(87% of the 54 successful groups)*

    7 groups were sole-led   *(13%)*

        Of the 14 planned groups which did not happen:

    5 groups were planned as sole-led   *(36% of groups not progressing beyond planning)*

The groupwork learners

122 learners took part in the Groupwork Project

  58 social work trained   *(48% of the total)*

  59 social care staff   *(48% of the total)*

    5 others   *4% of the total)*

  91 were involved in successful groups   *(75% of all learners)*

The groupwork portfolios

48 portfolios were submitted   *(39% of learners)*

  28 from social work trained staff   *(58% of portfolios)*

  20 from social care workers   *(42% of portfolios)*

  41 passed on first submission   *(85% of portfolios)*

    5 passed on re-submission   *(10% of portfolios)*

    2 were unsuccessful   *(4% of portfolios)*

31 different groups (57% of all groups which ran successfully) were represented in the 48 portfolios (many co-workers submitted their own portfolio around the same group)

All figures are correct as of 2005.

A generalist model of groupwork must, of course, take account of context. Indeed, the significance of the context in which groups and groupwork take place will be a strong and recurring theme in the book. Ironically, the significance of the specific context is, itself, a general and common characteristic to all groups and groupwork practice, and sits comfortably within a generalist model.

Documenting practice

This book is based on the learning derived not just from the nine illustrative groups, but from all the 54 groups in the Groupwork Project (Box 1.1) and, indeed, those 14 groups which were unsuccessful in moving from the planning stage. This learning has been amplified by the fact that 48 of the 122 participants in the project documented their groupwork learning and practice in a systematic and standardised format. To do this they used a portfolio: a collection of materials to demonstrate the learning and practice ability of its author (Doel and Shardlow, 1995). Portfolios have great potential to develop practice by availing the wider practice community of detailed information.

The groupwork portfolios provide particularly rich detail for the lives of 31 of the 54 groups in the project. Each portfolio was structured in the same way. Data were collected in a standardised format and systematically presented by the groupworkers, who were asked first to describe, then to analyse, and finally to reflect on 18 different aspects of the group and their own groupwork practice, thus providing over 50 sets of information. In addition, appendices in each portfolio provided direct materials from the group itself, as well as a video-tape of the group in session, when the appropriate permissions could be obtained.[1]

Although the idea of 'portfolio' goes beyond the conventional notion of a case or group record or even a groupwork 'assignment' (Wayne and Cohen, 2001), it is interesting to locate the groupwork portfolio in the broad history of social work documentation. For example, the understanding that documents can be used to construct and develop a common knowledge base for practice was demonstrated almost a century ago by Mary Richmond (1917). This involved social work practice rather than groupwork practice, but the premise that representations of practice (whether in case files or portfolios) can inform practice development has a long tradition. Shortly after Richmond's text, Ada Eliot Sheffield (1920) authored an entire book on case records, *Social Case History*. Most interesting of all for groupworkers is Grace Coyle's (1937) *Studies in Group Behaviour*, a book based on case studies of five groups. These groups had engaging names such as 'The Gay Girls', 'The Merry-Makers' and 'The Concordia Club – a study of hilarity and conflict'. Therefore, the process of using practitioners' documented work to inform and shape future professional practice has a long history (Gilbert, 2004).

The advantage of the groupwork portfolio is that it is written not as a case record but as a descriptive, analytical and reflective account of the practitioner's learning and practice development, with case material as illustration. For the purposes of exploring how groupwork is practised and how groupworkers conceptualise their practice, the portfolio is a better instrument than an agency case record. Any potential distortions arising from a portfolio author's desire to present their shiniest practice, were countered by a strong message from the Groupwork Project that some of the 'best' evidence comes from those times when the groupworker feels most challenged ('calm seas ne'er produce an able seaman'). In fact, the portfolios were, by and large, refreshingly candid, reflecting the honesty experienced in the workshops and consultations. (For more details about the training programme which supported the project, see Doel and Sawdon, 1999b.)

This book has grown out of the detailed reading and analysis of portfolios of groupwork practice and learning, so that the architecture of the book reflects the themes which arose from the practitioners' own groupwork. This has been a rewarding experience, which I hope will have a positive effect on the authenticity and relevance of what is presented.

Theorising from practice

The development of portfolios in recent years has made it possible to draw on practitioners' own words in a systematic way. Although writing about experiences helps them to 'become clearer and more objective for later study' (Lähteenmäki, 2005), this is only the case if the manner of the writing is accessible and systematic. If the learning is to become more than personal, broader than anecdotal, it needs to be sufficiently standardised to bear comparison and contrast with others recording their experiences, too. As Sheldon and MacDonald (forthcoming) note, 'Informed practitioners are potential contributors to the knowledge base, if they so organize their evaluations of their work that they are reliable enough to be fed back into the research and development process'.

The portfolio can provide an authentic window on how groupwork is experienced and practised, and the portfolio template is constructed in such a way as to peel away the groupworkers' thinking, so that we learn not just about what happens in the group, but how the groupworkers conceptualise this experience and how they learn from it. We have an insight into how individual groupworkers are conceptualising their own practice as 'insider-researchers' (McDermott, 2005) and this, in itself, is of immense value. However, can we go further and consider these conceptualisations as 'a collective experience'? In other words, are there ways in which we can use each individual portfolio as a brick which, together, construct a greater understanding? This book is something of an experiment, but hypothesises that the answer is probably 'yes'. If one portfolio provides evidence of the way in which an individual groupworker is theorising their practice, it seems reasonable to suggest that, taken together, we should be able to learn even more about how groupwork practice is theorised. Given the broad range of groups in the sample, we should also be able to learn more about the nature of the core elements of groupwork.

There are some cautions. First, the sample remains relatively small, even though it is large in comparison with what else is available. Certainly, there is a wide variety of groups, but they are all housed within one social work agency, a statutory social services department in northern England (with the exception of the Crimestop probation service group). They are all created groups, that is the groupworkers were responsible for their formation. None are user-led or self-help in nature. None are primarily social action groups (Ward, 2004; *Groupwork* journal, 2004). Second, all the 'bricks' have been fired in the same kiln; in other words, since all the groupworkers were trained through the one project, is it possible that we are merely looking at our own reflection? What we put in to the training is merely reflected back through the portfolios. There are, then, advantages and disadvantages to being an insider. This contrasts, say, with the groups with which Phillips (2001) illustrates her text, where she has the advantages and the disadvantages of being an outsider.

Third, the portfolios are instruments not just of learning and practice, but also of assessment (Doel *et al.*, 2002). Knowing that a judgement will be made on the basis of the portfolio, how tempered is the evidence presented by the portfolio authors? These, and no doubt other, factors all need to be taken into consideration before any larger claims can be made about the collective evidence to be derived from these portfolios of groupwork practice.

Of course, the portfolios are not the sole evidence. The wider experience of the project included workshops and consultations which provided a rounded picture, and we have a wealth of groupwork experience through the formal literature, though the evidence base is yet in its infancy (Preston-Shoot, 2004). We shall consider this in more detail in Chapter 9.

Unusually, then, this book takes its primary references from groupworkers' portfolios rather than traditional academic referencing.[2] The quotations in this book are taken direct from portfolios and only occasionally modified to clarify meaning. The number which follows each reference (e.g. Portfolio P, 5.2) is the relevant section in the portfolio, and 'P&O' is an abbreviation for 'Power and Oppression', a regular unit through the portfolio.

As well as the advantages and the innovations of this approach, there are also some difficulties. Practitioners' portfolios are somewhere between the private and the public domains, so I have respected the confidentiality of their authors and the reader is unable to visit the source. With quotations from published works you can follow up the sources directly, and judge for yourself how representative the quotations are. Until we have a systematic way of making practice experience available, perhaps in an electronic library available to all (with safeguards for the confidentiality of service users and carers), this kind of access is not possible. Nevertheless, I trust that the disadvantages are outweighed by the advantages, and I have attempted a faithful representation of the themes emerging from the groups as demonstrated in the portfolios. I hope that the unmediated voice of practitioners will become increasingly common as a principle reference.

Discovering how practitioners theorise is central to the development of practice, groupwork or otherwise. Chapters 2 and 9 will consider in more detail the basis for our current understanding of groups and groupwork, and how the evidence base might grow.

The nine groups

Nine groups illustrate the book. All were supported by the Groupwork Project training programme, and all but one were located in the same social services department ('Crimestop' was in a Probation Service). The groups could be referred to as case studies, but I prefer the notion of *storytelling*. The stories of these groups, their individual members and the groupworkers, are a powerful narrative which helps us to 'empathize with the experiences of others' (Fairbairn, 2002: 24). It is, after all, this ability to empathise with the narrative of these stories that helps us to make sense of our own experience and learning, and to make the translation into our own groupwork practice.

The groups have been chosen to reflect the variety of the project, but they are not intended in any way to be carefully representative. In some respects the choice of groups is immaterial, given the central premise of the book that groupwork has generic elements and that strong connecting themes link groupwork in contrasting situations. However, I recognise that, as the reader, you are likely to relate more to some of the group's contexts than others. Even so, a strong message from many of the participants in the project was the benefit derived from the opportunity to learn about groups in unfamiliar settings, alongside people in circumstances very different to those they usually encountered. Learning can accelerate when you cannot call on a stock response. This is useful advice for your progress through this book; when approaching the activities in each chapter, it can be useful to choose to work on examples in territory which is new to you.

Even where there seem to be stark differences between groups, such as the degree of choice which group members have regarding membership, we will see that these differences lie along the same continuum, rather than at unconnected, opposite poles. Learning about the notion of compulsion from studying a group where members are present because of a court order can tell us much about the nature of so-called 'choice' in groups where members are self-selected.

An outline of each of the nine groups is sketched in the boxes at the end of this chapter (Boxes 1.C to 1.W). You will be able to refer back to these profiles as you read the book. All names have been anonymised and a unique identifying letter is used for each group. For example, the Crimestop group is Group C, the names of the groupworker, co-workers and members all begin with C, and the portfolio reference is Portfolio C. I hope this will enable you to differentiate quickly between different groups as they appear in the text. The few quotations from portfolios not in this sample are referenced as Portfolio X and all boxes are numbered by taking the number of the chapter as the first number, so Box 3.2 is the second Box in Chapter 3.

The groupworkers and the group members

We see the groups through the eyes of the nine groupworkers. From their perspective we have a reasonably clear view of the group members, whose stories provide the fabric of the group. Groupworkers and group members are two of the 'drivers' identified by Preston-Shoot (2004: 23) when considering the search for evidence of groupwork's effectiveness. Like the groups themselves, the practitioners are not chosen to be strictly representative of the 122 learners who took part in the Groupwork Project, though they do reflect the range of participants. There are six social workers with varying years of post-qualifying experience, two social care workers without a social work qualification, and one probation officer. Eight of the nine are women, eight are white and one is dual heritage. They were located in various settings – adult services, community mental health, children's services (family support; child and adolescence mental health), family centre, leaving care project, youth offending and probation. All nine groupworkers had co-workers and there are occasional quotations from the portfolios of two of these co-workers.

I have described the access which portfolios give to the perspectives of groupworkers. It is possible to learn much about the group members, too. Group members' evaluations were included, and groupworkers were regularly asked to reflect on their participation and progress, both in terms of individual members and the group as a whole. Video recordings of some sessions provided a direct window into the group. However, with more resources it would have been desirable to discover members' views directly, rather than at one remove. Even so, the portfolios as a whole give us a systematic insight into the group experience of over two hundred people.

The group members of the nine groups with which you will become familiar reflect a wide range of people: women with mental health problems, older people with memory difficulties, young people who have offended, adult offenders, young people leaving the care of the local authority, carers, parents of children with behavioural difficulties, disadvantaged families in a local community. They are more female and more white than the general population, which reflects the profile of the group membership overall in the Project.

I was able to contact most of the groupworkers, all of whom were delighted that their groupwork learning would be shared with a wider audience. It was never a possibility that group members could be contacted, but all group members gave permission for their own and the group's story to be told in the pages of the groupworker's portfolio. Personal details, such as names, have remained anonymous and any specific identifying features have been removed.

INTRODUCING THE NINE GROUPS

Box 1.C   Crimestop (Portfolio C)
Box 1.F   Family Support (Portfolio F)
Box 1.H   Women of Hope (Portfolio H)
Box 1.J   Memory Joggers (Portfolio J)
Box 1.M   Managing Behaviour for Carers (Portfolio M)
Box 1.O   Offending Awareness (Portfolios O, O1)
Box 1.P   Parents Plus (Portfolios P, P1)
Box 1.S   Sound Start (Portfolio S)
Box 1.W   Westville Women (Portfolio W)

The outlines of the groups in Boxes 1.C to 1.W are taken directly from the groupworkers' portfolios. You will want to refer back to these as you read more about the groups during the course of the book.

KEY POINTS

▪ This book seeks to understand the common elements of 'groupwork' in very diverse settings and contexts.
▪ The book is an experiment in theorising from practice, using the systematic accounts of groupworkers to help develop a generalist understanding of groupwork.
▪ The book is underpinned by the documented experience of a Groupwork Project to develop groupwork in a mainstream social services department in northern England.
▪ Nine illustrative groups are used throughout the book.
▪ Some academic referencing is used in the book, but the primary reference point is the evidence from practitioners, with extensive quotations from portfolios of groupwork practice.

FURTHER READING

Doel, M., Sawdon, C. and Morrison, D. (2002) *Learning, Practice and Assessment: signposting the portfolio,* London: Jessica Kingsley,
This book considers the relationship between learning, practice and assessment, with especial reference to continuing professional development. It provides more detail concerning the Groupwork Project and the middle section of the book reproduces an entire Groupwork Portfolio.

Manor, O. (ed.) (2000) *Ripples: Groupwork in Different Settings,* London: Whiting and Birch.
A collection of articles edited by Oded Manor which, together, demonstrate the impressive range of groupwork practice.

Marsh, P. and Doel, M. (2005) *The Task-Centred Book,* London: Routledge/Community Care.
This book also uses practitioners' experience, as recorded in portfolios, as an evidence base for a social work practice method (in this case it is task-centred practice).

FOOTNOTES

1 The text of a complete groupwork portfolio is reproduced in Doel *et al.* (2002).
2 Also see *The Task-Centred Book* (Marsh and Doel, 2005), which documents a parallel Task-Centred Project in the same agency as the Groupwork Project.

BOX 1.C THE CRIMESTOP GROUP

(Portfolio C)

Main purpose of the group

To enhance male offenders' capacity to change in such a way that reduces the risk of their victimising other people.

Group leadership

Claire is a Probation Officer, qualified for four years, working in the Community Supervision team of a Probation service. Claire is white and in her late twenties. Claire has three co-workers on the Crimestop programme, two men and one woman, all white.

Group membership

Open or closed membership? *closed*
Number of members: *8*
Largest group attendance: *11;* Smallest attendance: *4;* Average attendance: *9*
Age range of group members: *25–56 years*

Box 1.C continued

Gender and ethnic composition: *all male, white British*
Voluntary or compulsory membership: *compulsory*

Group sessions

Where did/does the group meet? *a designated group room in the Probation Service premises*
How often? *3 mornings a week for 11 weeks*
How long is each session approximately? *2 1/2 hours, with break*
Open-ended or time-limited? *time-limited*
Any other details?
Group members attend as a condition of a Probation Order. Failure to do so may result in a return to Court where a custodial sentence is the ultimate sanction.

Pen pictures of two group members

Ceiran is a single white man aged around 30. He is on a one-year Probation Order with a requirement inserted to complete a group. This order was imposed for offences of commercial burglary which were motivated by the desire/need to fund alcohol use. His expectations of the group were minimal. He had a discussion with a former group member who had been breached and sent to prison as a result. Ceiran had expected the same to happen to him when he was breached for failure to report to the group, but the order was allowed to continue and Ceiran went on to complete the group. He is seen by the group as lazy and uncaring. At the end of the group his attitude had shifted only slightly and I believe he would have benefited more if he had started the group in the frame of mind in which he ended it.

Carl is a 40-year-old white man who is single, with contact with a daughter from a previous relationship. He never lived with his partner and contact is often interrupted by acrimony between the two. He is a senior group member who has been addicted to heroin for 20 years. His offence was possession of heroin. He is mature and thoughtful. He has some insight into his offending and a degree of motivation despite many 'failures'. Carl is bemused by a lot of the material [used in the group programme], and presents almost as if joining in is 'below' him, but once he commits himself he appears to enjoy it. He says on occasion that he is beyond help, but admits that the group meets his need for company as he is isolated. He presents as physically dirty sometimes and the group 'hold him at arm's length'. However, he wins them over with his thoughtful, intelligent contribution and supportive attitude.

BOX 1.F FIRWOOD FAMILY SUPPORT GROUP

(Portfolio F)

Main purpose of the group

To provide family support in the Firwood area, bringing families together for mutual support in a neutral and safe environment, reducing isolation and vulnerability. We aim to provide practical resources such as a toy library and a clothing exchange. Outside agencies are invited to offer advice on issues such as health, benefits, children's behaviour.

Group leadership

Fran is a qualified social worker in a Children and Families team. She is dual heritage. Her co-worker, Flora, is a social care manager (a pre-qualified worker). Formerly there were two other co-workers: Fiona and Filomena. Fiona was the Section Head and Filomena was a qualified social worker. Fiona and Filomena have moved on. Flora and Filomena are white and Fiona is black.

Group membership

Open or closed membership? *open*
Number of members: *8*
Largest group attendance: *14;* Smallest attendance: *3;* Average attendance: *6*
Age range of group members: *22 42 years*
Gender and ethnic composition: *7 white females and 1 white male*
Voluntary or compulsory membership: *voluntary*

Group sessions

Where did/does the group meet? *'The Centre', Firwood*
How often? *weekly*
How long is each session approximately? *3 hours, with lunch*
Open-ended or time-limited? *open-ended*
How long has the group been running? *18 months*

Pen pictures of two group members

Frank is white British and the only male to attend the group regularly. Frank is unemployed and has been since he hurt his back some years ago. I don't feel that Frank is 'intimidated' by being the only male in a predominantly female group; on the contrary, this rather encourages him in showing his 'manliness'.

Box 1.F continued

Frank can be quite loud and intimidating in his manner of speaking to people, and in some respects his non-verbal communication, and this may lead to him being quite oppressive with other group members. Frank also suffers from mental health problems. I feel Frank enjoys attending the group and finds support, this coming mainly from the group leaders as opposed to the members.

Fizz is recently married and has two children to her previous marriage; both have been diagnosed as having Attention Deficit and Hyperactivity Disorder (ADHD). Fizz can only be described as presenting everything as 'doom, gloom and despair'. She rarely has anything positive to say about anything or any situation and is persistently pessimistic.

   All this said, Fizz is an active participant in the group and becomes involved in many of the activities that are on offer. Although quite negative about her own children, who both attend school full time, she is very good with the other group members' children and displays patience and understanding with them.

BOX 1.H THE WOMEN OF HOPE GROUP

(Portfolio H)

Main purpose of the group

To promote, encourage and create an opportunity for individual women suffering from depression, anxiety and panic attacks to have a better understanding of their illness; initiate positive thinking; build self-esteem and confidence; develop communication and links with the community.

Group leadership

Helen *is a Senior Social Work practitioner, Community Mental Health team. She is a white woman.*
Her co-worker, **Harriet,** *is a Community Psychiatric Nurse.*

Group membership

Open or closed membership? *closed - adult women with severe and enduring mental health problems*
Number of members: 7
Largest group attendance: *7;* Smallest attendance: *3;* Average attendance: *6*
Age range of group members: *30–35 years*
Gender and ethnic composition: *white, female*
Voluntary or compulsory membership: *voluntary*

Box 1.H continued

Group sessions

Where did/does the group meet? *'The Clinic' at the CMHT centre*
How often? *weekly*
How long is each session approximately? *2 hours 15 minutes*
Open-ended or time-limited? *time-limited (10 sessions)*

Pen pictures of two group members

Hayley is aged 48, white European. She came to the group to meet with other females who had similar difficulties. She hoped to gain confidence and to be able to meet with others like herself. She attended 7 sessions out of the 10. She was perceived as a strong member of the group, fairly self-centred, she does have a good sense of humour, she has a tendency to monopolise. Hayley is married with a grown-up son.

Hazel is a 48-year-old single parent, white European, with two girls aged 10 and 16 living at home with her. She has grown-up sons and a grown-up daughter by a former marriage. She is perceived by the group as a quiet person, with little interaction. She came to the group because she rarely went out due to mental and physical ill-health. Hazel felt her life was so monotonous, she felt alone and isolated, despite a supportive family. She attended six sessions.

BOX 1.J THE MEMORY JOGGERS GROUP

(Portfolio J)
Main purpose of the group

To provide a quality service to men and women with mild to moderate dementia whose needs are not currently met in the local area.

Aims: to provide social contact to counter isolation; to offer stimulation to people's short- and long-term memories; to help maintain members' existing skills and learn new ones; to increase self-esteem and confidence by offering support, advice and encouragement; to help promote independence.

Group leadership

Jenny is a qualified social worker in a Community Mental Health team. Her co-worker, Jill, is also a social worker in the team, and two other groupworkers, Julie and Joy are mental health support workers.

Box 1.J continued

Group membership

Open or closed membership? *open*
Number of members: *11*
Largest group attendance: *11;* Smallest attendance: *6;* Average attendance: *8*
Age range of group members: *50–80+ years*
Gender and ethnic composition: *mainly women, white, working class backgrounds*
Voluntary or compulsory membership: *voluntary (though many members may be wanting to please family members or us, the group facilitators)*

Group sessions

Where did/does the group meet? *At first, the James Clinic, but this closed down, so then we moved to Jonesmoor Hospital.*
How often? *weekly, Monday afternoons*
How many sessions has the group had? *15*
How long is each session approximately? *2 hours*
Open-ended or time-limited? *open-ended*

Pen pictures of two group members

Jane is in her late 70s, lives with her husband in a ground floor flat, both having moved to Cityville some months ago to be near her son. I am Jane's social worker. She has had a long-term involvement with psychiatric services, but has always been reluctant to have any form of intervention from services. Jane was hesitant about attending but agreed to visit on a trial basis 'because you will be there' and has been a regular member ever since. For the first few weeks both she and her husband forgot about the group, but now it is a regular weekly feature. She participates well in group activities, especially arts and crafts. She is very good at memory games, especially with the use of prompt cards, but finds it difficult coming to terms with her memory deficits. When she can't remember she becomes quiet and sits back. Other members may say they can't remember but Jane doesn't. She doesn't participate. Over the months she has become more relaxed and formed good bonds with the other members.

Jim lives in sheltered accommodation. He is 77 years old and was referred by the local community team. Jim was quite a powerful member. His mood was unpredictable, one minute clowning about, the next moody and withdrawn. He has both long- and short-term memory problems. Jim needed close supervision and he would often misinterpret situations and go off at a tangent. He had a good rapport with the group facilitators and was a popular group member. Being an ex-boxer he has a physical presence which may have been threatening; however, that wasn't the case with the group. Others viewed him as comic, he was well-liked and accepted. Two members, in particular, seemed to have a calming effect on him. For many weeks he was a regular attender, although reluctant at times, requiring friendly persuasion, he would attend sessions and leave happy. However, it reached a stage when he refused to attend and became agitated when approached. Jim no longer attends the group but is still supported by a Community Psychiatric Nurse from our team.

BOX 1.M BEHAVIOUR MANAGEMENT GROUP

(Portfolio M)

Main purpose of the group

To bring together a small group of people who are or will be caring for children under the age of 8, to build on existing skills and learn tactics and strategies for dealing with challenging behaviour.

Group leadership

Mandy *is a white woman in her early 40s, working as a Family Worker in the Middletown Family Centre. Her co-worker,* **Meg***, is also a white woman in her early 40s, working as a Family Worker in the Middletown Family Centre. Mandy and Meg do not have a professional qualification.*

Group membership

Open or closed membership? *closed*
Number of members: *8*
Largest group attendance: *8;* Smallest attendance: *6;* Average attendance: *7*
Age range of group members: *29–43 years*
Gender and ethnic composition: *7 white females and 1 black female*
Voluntary or compulsory membership: *voluntary*

Group sessions

Where did/does the group meet? *Middletown Family Centre*
How often? *7 sessions over 14 weeks (4 sessions; 5-week break; 2 sessions; 2-week break; final follow-up session)*
How long is each session approximately? *2 hours*
Open-ended or time-limited? *time-limited*
Any additional notes? *We arranged for a crèche and this was very important in enabling group members to attend.*

Pen pictures of three group members

Marcia is aged 43 and is a black female. She wants to gain 'as much information as possible and shared experience'. Marcia has been fostering for 8 years and has cared for 42 children on short-term placement during that time. She has teenage children of her own and is fostering a 4-month-old baby at the moment. Marcia is also a registered child minder, day carer and pre-adoptive carer. Marcia is reserved but obviously has a lot of experience and good sound advice to offer the group. She has a good sense of humour and comes over as a leader who people can look up to and respect.

Box 1.M continued

Moira is aged 38 and is a white female. She wants to meet with other carers and in her own words 'to get ideas'. Moira is very new to fostering and her first placement is a 7-year-old boy who has been diagnosed as having Attention Deficit Hyperactivity Disorder (ADHD). This seems a challenging first placement which could possibly break down. Moira has three children of her own aged between 8 and 14 years. She is also a registered childminder. Moira appears quiet, very nervous and unsure, reluctant to speak out and in need of support and advice. She leans on Molly (her sister-in-law) for some of this support.

Molly is aged 35 and is a white female. She wants to understand more about other children. Molly has been fostering for nine months, short-term and emergency placement. She recently had a placement of three siblings which broke down. Molly now fosters one 10-month-old girl. She has three children of her own aged between 3 and 14 years. Molly appears talkative, confident and 'loud', though not in an offensive way. As she is new to fostering she will gain from the support of the other carers and gain new ideas from the group.

BOX 1.O OFFENDING AWARENESS GROUP

(Portfolios O and O1)

Main purpose of the group

To promote awareness and provoke thought and discussion surrounding issues relevant to a young person's offending behaviour.

Group leadership

Orla is a 24-year-old white woman, a graduate but not qualified professionally. She works in a Youth Offending Team, with the Intensive Supervision and Surveillance Programme (ISSP), a community punishment scheme which aims to reduce re-offending. Young people aged 10–17 can be sentenced by the courts to the scheme for six months. The first three months is intense (minimum of 25 hours contact each week), with a minimum of 7 hours supervision in the second three months.

*Her main co-worker, **Oliver**, is a 31-year-old white male, also an ISSP worker and a newly qualified social worker. Orla has three other co-workers.*

Box 1.0 continued

Group membership

Open or closed membership? *Open; young people are regularly referred by the courts, so the group may gain new members and lose them, but with the hope for some continuity of membership.*
Number of members: *varies*
Largest group attendance: *10;* Smallest attendance: *3;* Average attendance: *4–6*
Age range of group members: *14–17 years (potentially 10–18 years)*
Gender and ethnic composition: *so far, all male, though potential for young women; predominantly white reflecting the ethnic composition of the catchment area*
Voluntary or compulsory membership: *compulsory (Community Order of the court), facing breach proceedings if not valid justification for absence*

Group sessions

Where does the group meet? *Youth Offending Team premises in the town centre*
How often? *The group is on-going every Monday and Wednesday; it is expected that each young person will attend 2 sessions per week for 10 weeks (20 sessions).*
How long is each session approximately? *2 hours*
Open-ended or time-limited? *open-ended; 10-week membership for each individual*

Pen pictures of three group members

Oz is aged 15 years and is white, the first young person to be sentenced to the programme. As Oz is now onto the less intensive stage of the programme, he will only attend occasional groupwork sessions, as deemed appropriate by me and his caseworker. He completed much of the work to be covered in the group during individual sessions before the group programme was up and running. Oz is very intelligent and perceptive and can present opinions well when he feels strongly about an issue. He can be disruptive at times and attempts to dominate.

O'Connor is aged 17 and white and recently joined the programme, so will be expected to attend all sessions as he has had no prior individual work in any area. O'Connor has minor learning difficulties. To compensate for this, O'Connor sometimes takes on the role of 'entertainer'.

Owen is aged 17, white, and currently on his less intensive phase of the programme and so will attend only certain relevant sessions. Other members of the group may feel able to bully Owen, as he is generally low in confidence and not as perceptive as many of the others. Owen also struggles with concentration for any long period of time.

BOX 1.P PARENTS PLUS GROUP

(Portfolios P and P1)

Main purpose of the group

To provide a programme aimed at facilitating better communication between parents and young people aged 11–14 years.

Group leadership

Paul *is Principal Social Worker, Child and Adolescence Mental Health Team. His co-worker,* **Petra***, is a social worker with the Family Support Team. Both Paul and Petra are white, as is the membership of the group.*

Group membership

Open or closed membership? *closed, although new members missing only one or two sessions might attend*
Number of members: *4*
Largest group attendance: *4;* Smallest attendance: *1;* Average attendance: *2*
Age range of group members: *31–47 years*
Gender and ethnic composition: *female, white British*
Voluntary or compulsory membership: *voluntary*

Group sessions

Where did/does the group meet? *Pathways community centre*
How often? *weekly*
How long is each session approximately? *2 hours*
Open-ended or time-limited? *time-limited – 8 sessions*

Pen pictures of two group members

Penny is aged 38. She was invited to join the group initially as a result of being identified as a parent on the CAMHS* waiting list who may wish to join a group. Attended on the first occasion with her partner, Phil, from whom she is separated, and up to week 6 had attended every session. Phil only attended week 1, we were given to believe to support Penny. The mother of two daughters, Penny holds down a responsible job and is articulate and thoughtful. Her chosen style of parenting is based on rational negotiation. The younger of her two daughters, Petal, presented Penny with considerable difficulties. Her older daughter, Poppy, moved out to live with her father Phil. Penny was prepared to give the group a try despite not expecting to learn anything new.

* Childhood and Adolescence Mental Health Service

Box 1.P continued

Pat is aged 39. Her son, Peter (12) had been referred to CAMHS with 'behavioural difficulties'. Pat is a single carer with an older daughter, and a younger niece living at home. The niece is subject to a Residence Order. Pat is not employed and has only recently returned to her home area and extended family, having lived in the south of England for a number of years. Her husband still lives in the south and contact with the children is an area of difficulty. From the outset, Pat has been enthusiastic about the group and has used some of the suggested approaches effectively. She can be less aware of the impact her often extended anecdotes can have on others waiting to make their contribution.

BOX 1.S SOUND START GROUP

(Portfolio S)

Main purpose of the group

To provide a realistic concept of options for moving on and procedures;
To build self-confidence through opportunities to share ideas in the group;
To alleviate fears of moving on.

Group leadership

Samantha is a Project Worker in a Leaving Care team, working with 16–21-year-olds to prepare them for independence after they leave care. She is recently qualified. Other workers in the project involved in the group are Sonia, Steve, Sally, Suzy and Shana. They are all white.

Group membership

Open or closed membership? *closed*
Number of members: 6
Largest group attendance: *6;* Smallest attendance: *3;* Average attendance: *4*
Age range of group members: *16–17 years*
Gender and ethnic composition: *all White British; 1 male and 5 females*
Voluntary or compulsory membership: *voluntary, though an expectation that all newly registered young people attend this group*

Group sessions

Where did/does the group meet? *basement room of the Project Centre*

Box 1.S continued

How often? *twice weekly for 6 sessions (3 weeks)*
How long is each session approximately? *2 hours*
Open-ended or time-limited? *time-limited*

Pen pictures of two group members

Stacey is a white 17-year-old. She comes to the group because she wants to and also her foster carer strongly encourages her. Stacey hoped to find out about accommodation options when she moved on. Her friend, Sharleen, attends. Stacey has attended the group even when it has had to be postponed! Stacey is seen as Sharleen's other half as they always sit together. Stacey has arrived at the group on a couple of occasions in a silent mood due to disagreements at home. Her reluctance to join in and her downcast mood confuse the group and they try to be sensitive and inclusive. Stacey has used this to become the centre of attention in quite a manipulative way.

Simon is a white 16-year-old. He is the only male in the group. He attends because he is encouraged to do so by his social worker and because he gets on well with the rest of the group. The social side of the group seems to be more important to Simon than the idea of moving on [from care to independent living]. He attends regularly and missed two sessions because he did not receive the message that it was happening. The group see Simon as very loud and boisterous. They respond positively to him, in terms of laughing at jokes when he is present, but when he is absent they talk quite negatively about how loud he is.

BOX 1.W WESTVILLE WOMEN'S GROUP

(Portfolio W)

Main purpose of the group

a) To offer a group experience for women who, because of their particular mental health needs, are typically not offered this type of opportunity.
b) To promote self-confidence and esteem.
c) To promote greater understanding of mental health issues as relating to women.

Group leadership

Wendy *is a white social worker in Westville Community Mental Health team. Her co-worker,* **Win,** *is a social work assistant. The team is multi-disciplinary.*

(also see Box 2.3, page 36)

Box 1.W continued

Group membership

Open or closed membership? *closed*
Number of members: 6
Largest group attendance: 6; Smallest attendance: 3; Average attendance: 5
Age range of group members: *34–58 years*
Gender and ethnic composition: *all white females*
Voluntary or compulsory membership: *voluntary*

Group sessions

Where did/does the group meet? *Westville Health Centre*
How often? *weekly for 10 sessions*
How long is each session approximately? *1.5 hours (there have been 2 half-days)*
Open-ended or time-limited? *time-limited*

Pen pictures of two group members

Wanda is a 39-year-old white woman who has a diagnosis of schizophrenia. In a group setting, she appears quiet and timid and has quite severe shaking due to side-effects of medication. Some of the other group members also remember Wanda from a number of years ago when she lived on the streets. Because of these facts, the rest of the group tend to be quite protective of her, but also to see her as 'worse than me'. In fact, when given the chance, Wanda can be very assertive. She came to the group to try something new, and was especially keen to take part in the activity days. She came to all the sessions apart from one, when she was on holiday.

Winsom is a 34-year-old white woman who was diagnosed as having a paranoid psychosis some time ago, requiring subsequent specialist support. She also sustained a head injury twelve years ago which resulted in some right-side paralysis which restricts her movement. She is fairly quiet in the group and does not give her opinion freely, although she is accepted. Winsom was curious to try out new activities and methods of dealing with mental health problems and has attended all sessions.

CHAPTER 2

UNDERSTAND

OBJECTIVES

By the end of this chapter you should:

▒ Understand the different elements in groups and groupwork practice

▒ Be aware of the range and kinds of knowledge that contribute to groupwork

▒ Connect groupwork practice to underpinning disciplines, such as philosophy

▒ Understand the range of systems which have an impact on groupwork

▒ Be aware of the ethical context for groupwork.

UNDERSTANDING GROUPWORK

> Whether some problem situations best lend themselves to a search for solutions in a group is a matter not yet fully resolved.
>
> Garvin *et al.*, 2004: 2

Conceptualisations of groupwork

If we take an example of a method of practice, we are likely to find that it can be used in either a group or an individual context. For example, task-centred groupwork and task-centred casework follow common task-centred principles and practice. The difference between task-centred groupwork and task-centred casework is, not unsurprisingly, the *groupwork*. We know what separates task-centred and cognitive behavioural models of practice, but what is it that unites task-centred *groupwork* and cognitive behavioural *groupwork?* What is the groupwork that they have in common? Understanding what it is that constitutes this groupwork is very much what this book is about. When we conceptualise groupwork, therefore, there are at least two dimensions along which models must be judged; the first is the appropriateness of the *practice model* (task-centred, cognitive-behavioural, etc.) and the second is the appropriateness of the *group context*.

One notion which is central to all practice methods in whatever context is that of *purpose*. The guiding principle of purpose is evident in the social goals, remedial and reciprocal models of Papell and Rothman (1968) and in Brown's (1994) seven group types. More recently, Garvin *et al.* (2004) have suggested these possible purposes for groupwork: enhancing individual function, enriching people's lives, ameliorating problems experienced by organisations and communities, producing social change and promoting social justice. In addition to purpose, groups have also been strongly characterised by the notion of developmental sequences, such as forming, storming, norming, performing and adjourning (Tuckman, 1965; Tuckman and Jensen, 1977) and Manor's (2000a) engagement, empowerment, mutuality and termination phases.

All of these models are ideal-types, and most, perhaps all, groups combine many kinds of purpose, and are not so much a series of steps and stages as a sense of emerging 'groupness', the erratic development of shared meanings and understandings. The real life of the group is much more complex than the two dimensions of any one model can suggest. Indeed, categories can create unhelpful boundaries without necessarily increasing understanding. As Garvin *et al.* (2004: 91) note, 'practice has become too eclectic to permit a neat typology of group work models'.

It is perhaps more helpful to consider the *profile* of a group, and to see this as composed of different elements (Box 2.1). Experience from the Groupwork Project (Box 1.1) suggests that the messy reality of experience is indeed best reflected not so much in discrete models or stages of groupwork, but in a consideration of these core elements. All groups embrace some of these elements, though they are found in differing degrees from group to group, each with its own unique 'fingerprint' composed of different degrees of each element (Box 2.2). So, it is not so much a question of which model to choose, but what hybrid is suggested by the particular elements of groupwork present in any one group. This gives rise not to discrete models of practice, but to complex patterns which will require much more research before we can make any definitive statements about the most effective combinations.

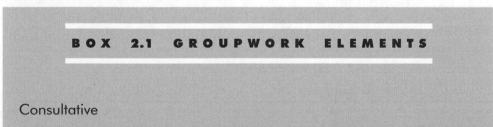

BOX 2.1 GROUPWORK ELEMENTS

Consultative

Facilitating group members to gain a better understanding of problems, opportunities, processes. The groupworker may be asked to work with an existing team or group to influence performance or working practices.

Box 2.1 continued

Educational

Teaching group members to learn new skills, attitudes and behaviours, often through cognitive activities. The groupworker introduces a variety of different learning styles into the group and monitors changes in individuals' abilities.

Social Action

Empowering group members to effect change in their environment, often with a campaigning element. The group is less likely to have a formal leader, and may be a self-help group, with professional assistance to access resources.

Social Control

Containing group members, perhaps by providing an alternative to harsher forms of social control. The groupworker helps mediate between the group and the authorities, aiming to reform individuals' behaviours and beliefs.

Social Support

Supporting group members to help maintain or improve their social functioning. The groupworker finds practical ways of bringing people together who may be isolated and to help them to develop mutual aid, perhaps becoming self-help.

Task

Enabling group members to achieve certain goals by developing and completing appropriate tasks. The groupworker helps the group to focus on its end-goal, suggests role allocations in the group and keeps the group alert to time limits.

Therapeutic

Helping group members to come to terms with past or current difficulties, often focusing on psychological issues such as trauma. The groupworker takes care of the group, assisting members to support each other to express their emotions.

We must also take account of the immense range of settings in which groupwork occurs. Even within one agency, groupwork can have an impressive presence, across community, residential and day settings, and with people from various social groups and in very different circumstances (see Box 1.1). In some circumstances, such as group care and group living, the group is its own community.

ACTIVITY 2.1: FINGERPRINTING

- In the introductory chapter we presented an outline for each of the groups used to illustrate this book. Consider the outlines for the Crimestop group (C), the Family Support group (F) and the Memory Joggers group (J), and for each of these three groups construct a likely *fingerprint*, in the manner of the Westville Women's group (W) in Box 2.2.
- If you are currently involved in a group, draw its fingerprint and consider the likely implications for the content and style of the group. You will find it useful to return to this as you read through this book.

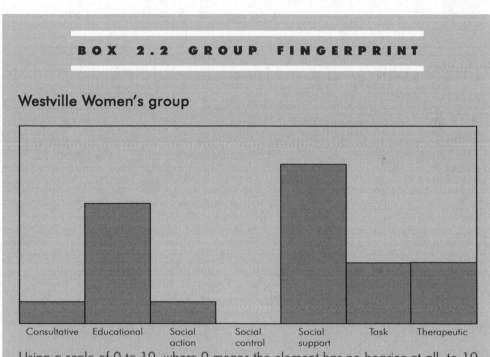

BOX 2.2 GROUP FINGERPRINT

Westville Women's group

Using a scale of 0 to 10, where 0 means the element has no bearing at all, to 10 which means it is very heavily present in the group, it is possible to develop a rough and ready 'fingerprint' for each group. The example above is the fingerprint for the Westville Women's group.

If we take the example fingerprint in Box 2.2, we see that the dominant elements are identified as educational and social support, whilst social control is absent and the consultative and social action elements are considered insignificant. What implications does this particular fingerprint have for the kind of groupwork which would best suit this group? To be honest, we have very little empirical evidence to guide the groupworker's plans. That is the bad news. The good news is that, whilst there can indeed be no one model of groupwork, there are universal groupwork principles and practices which promote good practice whatever the group's fingerprint, and that although the particular dilemmas which groupworkers face are experienced as very particular to the specific group, there are commonalities which enable you to transfer learning from one group experience to another, even when there are very different purposes.

Garvin *et al.* (2004: 5) state unequivocally that 'group work with an open-ended group is not the same as group work with a closed group. Group work on the computer is not the same as group work face-to-face'. They use this to argue for the need for theoretical specificity, though later recognise that there is an art to the application of practice guidelines. However, groupwork with one closed group can be very different from groupwork with another closed group, so we have to be careful that this logic does not reduce us to such levels of specificity that we can no longer understand 'groupwork'. Rather than looking for elusively precise practice principles, perhaps we need to understand better what makes groupwork *groupwork*. Essentially, that is the central purpose of this book.

Understanding the need (or not) for groupwork

Often it is our own experience which suggests the need for groupwork. This is a good basis to start, but we need to check this out; is our experience shared by others and do we know that this need is not being met elsewhere? Why do we think that groupwork is the best way to meet this need, and how can it be brought to the attention of our agency, perhaps via a planning group? (See Chapter 3.) The groupwork service will need to be proposed in a way which fits the agency's other provision. For example, the referral criteria which were developed for the Memory Joggers group (Box 1.J) made clear the gap in service which the group was intended to fill:

> This is a group for people with dementia who live in the Jamestown area. The group is aimed at people whose mental health needs cannot be met by the Johnson Resource Centre [a general day care service for older people], but who do not need the intensive support of The Junipers [for people with severe dementia]. There are currently no other day services in the Jamestown area for people with these needs, so the group aims to fill this gap in the service provision.
>
> Portfolio J, 2.1

Teams where there is a culture of sharing work experiences and reflecting on them can develop an awareness of service users with common needs. Wendy and her co-worker, Win, specifically wanted to include women with long-term severe mental illness because they were generally excluded from groupwork activities (Box 1.W).

> The initial idea for the group came out of recognition that a number of women on the team's caseloads had several similarities in terms of unmet needs. For example:
>
> 1 they had talked about how their illness had affected their confidence and self-esteem;
> 2 they had talked about loneliness and problems they had keeping a conversation alive;

3 they appeared to have poor understanding of their mental illness and little knowledge of alternative ways of helping outside traditional medication.

Portfolio W, 2.1

An organisation might understand groupwork to be an efficient way of managing the amount of work, as Fran notes below. This is fine as long as groupwork *is* the best way to meet the service users' needs, and the agency also accounts for the time needed to prepare and debrief from groups as well as the direct contact time in the group.

There was a large amount of family support work cases within the Firwood team and it was felt that a parenting support group could reduce the workload of individual social workers quite significantly.

Portfolio F, 2.1

Despite your desire to do groupwork, the local research might conclude that groupwork is not possible or appropriate. Often this is because there are insufficient numbers of people who are compatible, but it may be that needs are better met on an individual basis. If a group would be justified but there are not the resources, this information needs logging so that the potential group can have a call on resources if and when they do become available.

Knowledge for groupwork

We know relatively little about the different types of knowledge which social workers draw on in their practice (Sheppard *et al.*, 2001) and this is true for their groupwork practice, too. Lewis' (2002) formulation that *knowledge = evidence from research + practice wisdom + service user and carer experiences and wishes* is a useful one; for our purposes, 'service users and carers' = group members. This book's starting point is the second factor in Lewis' equation, 'practice wisdom'; however, we saw in Chapter 1 how collecting this wisdom in standardised ways and reflecting on it systematically can begin to transform the wisdom into 'evidence from research'. We also saw how the group members' voice can be amplified through the practitioners' documentation of experience in their groupwork portfolios.

The practitioners in the Groupwork Project (Box 1.1) had the advantage of making immediate use of the knowledge from the training workshops. It is likely that application of knowledge was assisted by its nearness in time and space – 'proximate' knowledge. These groupworkers were also generating new knowledge through their practice and bringing this back into the project via consultations and workshops, which in turn assisted them in making this knowledge more explicit. As Eraut (2005: 2) notes, 'the role of tacit knowledge in routinized professional practice is greatly underestimated, if not denied'. Groupwork can be a way of breaking out of this kind of routine, and over half (48) of the 91 learners who had the opportunity to practise groupwork recorded their practice systematically in a common portfolio format, where they also collected reflections on their learning. The knowledge from all of these experiences underpins this book.

An especially attractive feature of groupwork is its capacity to position group members' knowledge at the heart of professional practice. This knowledge, derived from the direct experience of service users and carers as group members, is too often neglected and subjugated (Croft and Beresford, 2002). It is much more difficult to neglect in groups, even in those which are heavily led and tightly scripted. The mathematics of a group (usually many more group members than groupworkers) and the central mission of groupwork, means that service user experience is inevitably a deep and essential resource, the very reason for bringing people together in the first place.

What constitutes knowledge has long been recognised as highly contested (Trevithick, 2005) and the knowledge of marginalised groups in society, such as service users, and black and ethnic minority groups, is often not heard, not counted and not valued. Groupwork is one way in which the current rhetoric about listening to service users and carers can become a reality. Groupwork practice has a rich tradition of listening to and acting on the voice of people whose knowledge has been considered peripheral, and of helping people to motivate and mobilise. There is still a long journey to find ways to disseminate this experiential knowledge, though the growing user-led research movement is showing the way. In addition to the different and unequal power bases of these sources of knowledge, they use such different languages and respect such different criteria that it is hard to overemphasise the challenge of bringing these together. This book is intended to be one small contribution.

Increasingly, there are attempts to codify and gather knowledge in social care in 'knowledge reviews' which are underpinned by the notion of the *quality* of knowledge and developing a better understanding of how knowledge works in social care (Pawson *et al.* 2003; Shaw *et al.,* 2004). For instance, an anecdote may be very illuminating, but we should be cautious about drawing any general conclusions from it. The beliefs and experiences of particular group members constitute very real truths for them, but might be at distinct odds from the truths for other group members. We also need to beware the creation of such tight criteria for knowledge that it is pushed far out of the reach of anybody without an enormous research budget to conduct randomised control trials (RCT). Indeed, there has been no large-scale RCT undertaken in the UK in social work overall, never mind groupwork specifically. Disentangling all the variables is extraordinarily complex. For example, though cognitive behaviour treatment (CBT) has 'significantly positive results against comparisons with either no intervention or with other commonly employed methods' (Sheldon, 2000: 70), how much is due to the CBT and how much is due to the groupwork in which CBT is frequently conducted? (Rose, 2004).

Topic-related knowledge

In addition to knowledge of groupwork, the worker needs knowledge and theoretical understanding around the content of the group. For example, if the group's purpose is to help people who misuse drugs and alcohol, groupworkers should have an understanding of substance misuse. Jenny might review Rishty's (2000) strengths perspective in reminiscence groupwork with depressed older adults to prepare for the Memory Joggers group. Paul, co-leading the Parents Plus group (Box 1.P) relates one of the member's success stories to his understanding of how the changes might be explained:

> Pat's story is in line with evidence about how [these changes] work: parents 'develop a belief system in which the child's difficult behaviour is attributed

to external situational circumstances rather than to intrinsic characteristics of the child' (Carr, 2000: 33).

Portfolio P, 7.2

The child of Penny, another member of this group, was assessed as possibly showing early indications of some form of disorder, which meant they were of a different order than her peers and the usual parenting techniques would have less effect. Understanding these differences is important to successful groupwork.

'Connecting' knowledge is important to relate one area, such as social work practice, to another, groupwork. Orla, the groupworker with the Offending Awareness group (Box 1.O), is aware that groupwork programmes have been shown to reduce offending behaviour by between 10% and 20% (Dixon, 2000: 14). Researching sessions around victim awareness, she also understands that the young offenders may have been victims themselves, and that there are many potential advantages to the group context.

> As Harrower (1993: 234) points out, 'groupwork with young offenders has particular advantages over traditional one-to-one casework. It allows those who are not adept at communicating, either verbally or non-verbally, to participate at their own level of expression and learn from observing others'.
>
> Portfolio O, 2.1

There are, then, at least three kinds of relevant knowledge and literature:

- The general groupwork literature (of which this book is an example);
- Context-specific literature, for example, relating to work with children, mental health work, criminal justice, working with older people;
- Specialist group methods, such as cognitive behavioural groupwork.

Where the group is part of a specific programme, there might be a ready-made supporting literature, which brings all of these components together. This was the case for Claire and the Crimestop group (Box 1.C). However, preparing for groupwork 'from scratch' requires a willingness to search widely.

ACTIVITY 2.2: SEARCHING

To prepare for the Westville Women's group for women with severe and enduring mental health problems, Wendy searched the following literature:

- General groupwork
- Feminist groupwork
- Groups for people experiencing mental illness
- Anti-oppressive social work
- Activity resources for women's mental well-being groups.

Take three of the groups outlined in Boxes 1.C to 1.W and consider what different areas of knowledge you would need to search in order to prepare for leadership

of the group. You should complete this activity with regard to any group you are
preparing to lead.

Groupwork and relevant disciplines

In this section I will look very briefly at examples of the way in which many different
disciplines contribute to our understanding of groupwork.

Philosophy

My focus is the existential aspect of groupwork, though there are many other branches
of philosophy. Groups can bring not just a sense of belonging, but a deeper sense of
meaning. Baggini (2004) explains that large and awkward existential questions such as
'what is the meaning of life?' can have either backward-reaching or forward-looking
responses. This is a useful insight for groupwork. For example, some groups may bring
meaning to its members by helping them consider, or re-consider, the past. The effects
of past, perhaps traumatic, experiences and a greater understanding of them might help
the group members to live more contentedly in the present. Although group members
will rarely have lived these past experiences with each other, they may discover that
there are similarities and that the consequences of these experiences are familiar.
Moreover, the group gives the opportunity to share the process of re-discovery and
assimilation.

Yet again, groups might seek meaning from forward-looking explanations. What
future purpose or goals will help give meaning to the group members? These may be
shared or related goals, or individuals in the group might share the process of determining
their own different meanings together. The group might well become an instrument by
which this forward-looking meaning can be achieved. Groupworkers may hold a tacit
belief that the group's meaning must come *either* from a backward-looking *or* from a
forward-looking orientation, whereas the group might best be served by combining
both kinds of meaning. Indeed, not everything has to be a means to an end; the group
might derive satisfaction just from *being*. This is neither backward nor forward, but
present. A combination of all three is likely to provide the deepest and most fulfilling
sense of meaning and value for the group. Chapters 4 and 5, in particular, consider
ways to develop meaningfulness and identity.

Politics

There are many levels at which politics and groupwork connect. Small groupwork
might be viewed as a training for participation in a social democracy, with mutual aid
models reflecting democratic ideals (Gitterman, 2004) and developing 'active citizenship'
(Silverlock, 2000). Certainly, groupwork is a practical expression of the ideology of
collective solutions, though there is a tension between the individualist, liberal values
which inform much social work, and the collective principles which inform both social
democracy and community work practice (Jordan, 2004). Groupworkers should reflect
on whether they believe their practice to focus on managing social problems and

containing social needs; or, alternatively, on 'transformational perspectives, geared not only to meeting social needs, but also addressing the causes of oppression and discrimination' (Mayo 1997: 169). Beliefs are underpinned by ideological assumptions and it is interesting to speculate whether the group as a context is ideologically neutral. A group can, for example, be used for social control as easily as social support, and both at the same time. Group pressure can be oppressive as well as liberating, and a commitment to groupwork can spring from an ideology of radicalisation or social conformity.

Issues of power are likely to be more transparent in groupwork, and none more so than the politics of gender (Cohen and Mullender, 2003). At a theoretical level, the dominant postmodern paradigm suggests that notions of 'male' and 'female' are simplistic, and that the divisions and subgroups within these categories are considerable. However, experience tells us that gender remains a significant element in the dynamics of groups, reflected in the continuing popularity of single gender groups, often using gender to define the group's title, as in the Women's group. The co-workers in the Women's group (Box 1.W) decided to exclude men from membership because they felt it less risky for women to be with one another, and to build trust more easily. It also prevents women from adopting stereotypical roles of deference to men (Portfolio W, 2.1). As Claire noted in respect of the offenders in the all-male Crimestop group:

> They tend not to ask a male colleague such questions as *'are you married?'*
> Portfolio C, 2.1

Most important is to remain open to all experiences of gender and not to deny a person's own experience of their gender because it does not fit our theories or beliefs. In many ways, this is no less than *the* groupwork challenge: to find commonalities whilst not denying differences. This theme runs throughout the book and is highlighted in Chapter 6.

Social and organisational psychology

One of the best known contributions to our knowledge of groupwork from social psychology is the concept of group pressure, made popular by a number of high-profile experiments (Asch, 1952). However, in this brief section I will highlight an element which is core to successful groupwork, difficult to establish in individual work, and often not considered explicitly: play and playfulness. The significance of play for children is well rehearsed, even though it is sometimes lacking in their lives (Simmond, 2005). Children generally have more opportunities for play in their everyday world, but the group may open up new kinds of play in which they can explore different aspects of their 'self'.

For adults, groups can provide permission for play, in all its many meanings. It may be a chance to play in the sense of have fun; the group might be the only place where some members are able to experience their 'child'. In addition, the group can be a place to play other roles, either formally in some kind of rehearsal of a situation to practise for the world outside, or implicitly by trying on new kinds of role – for instance, of one who helps rather than one who has been used to being helped. Playfulness is a significant part of being human and even in groups with painful and intense purposes, we should always find reasons for some playfulness. Chapter 5, in particular, considers ways in which groups can find their playfulness.

Cultures and structures in organisations have a direct impact on the delivery of services and they can be friendly or hostile towards groupwork as a mode of delivery. There are 'micro-climates', too, which influence the likelihood of groupwork taking root in this team or unit and not in that. A very useful concept from organisational psychology is that of the 'champion'. Chapter 9 considers the organisational context in greater detail and the significance of champions for groupwork.

Understanding ethical groupwork

> Central to social work practice with groups is the concept of mutual aid. The group worker recognizes that the group, with its multiple helping relationships, is the primary source of change. The group worker's role is one primarily of helping members work together to achieve the goals that they have established for themselves.
>
> (Association for the Advancement of Social Work with Groups [AASWG], 1999)

This statement introduces a set of 'Standards for Social Work Practice with Groups'. Behind the factual nature of the statements are ethical considerations about what groupwork *ought* to look like. Rightly or wrongly, these Standards would bring into question the legitimacy of groups where social control is a significant element, where membership is obligatory or even where content is prescribed by a manual. What we are reminded of is the moral purposes of groupwork and that groups are, themselves, moral agents. Groupwork is as much about helping a group to articulate a set of values as it is about learning new behaviours, sharing painful stories or achieving mutual goals.

The sharp end of ethical practice is, without doubt, groupwork by compulsion. The obligatory nature of the sessions of the Offending Awareness group (Box 1.O) raised particular ethical and practical issues for groupworker, Orla. As an alternative to custody, the group would probably be seen as a more positive option, though the compulsory nature of the group meant that non-attendance carried serious consequences, i.e. a decision to breach and removal of the young person to custody. Nevertheless, we can see that obligation can turn into fulfilment, and that there are often many constraints on 'free choice' (see Chapter 4 for more discussion on this topic).

> Despite initial protestations about attending, most of the young people began to view groupwork sessions as a welcome change from the individual work that had previously constituted much of their programme.
>
> Portfolio O, 3.2

Indeed, 'there are issues that are unique to ethical practice with groups' (Garvin *et al.* 2004: 2), not least the question of privacy and confidentiality, but also the obligation to reach out to populations who are often at the margins and who may be side-lined by the mainstream services. Ethical considerations are especially transparent for groupworkers because of the semi-public nature of a group. Power can be magnified in groups and this puts a particular onus on groupworkers to use their own power ethically to empower the group. Finally, the onus to evaluate the experience of the group is especially strong and complex for groupworkers, given the range of dynamics and systems involved. In Chapter 7 we will consider how value and values can be weighed with and by groups.

UNDERSTANDING GROUPS

Knowledge is one thing, understanding is another. We can know that $2 + 2 = 4$, but not understand why. We may not *know* what $4 + 4 =$, but if we understand why $2 + 2 = 4$, we can begin to discover what $4 + 4 =$. Understanding, not knowledge alone, is the key to effective professional practice, groupwork or otherwise.

One way to understand a group is to conceive it in terms of a number of different systems, all of which have an impact on the way it functions. Systems theories vary in the way they seek to explain how these systems interact and in this section we will use a notion of inner and outer systems; the best practice arises from a holistic understanding of all these systems (Doel *et al.*, 2002).

Inner systems

Understanding yourself

A significant element in the group system is yourself. This 'self' is a third addition to Schwartz's (1961) classic idea of the two clients – the individual members and the group as a whole. There are several reasons why it is important to have self-knowledge. First, is the significance of personal beliefs. These play an important part in the way in which knowledge is used or ignored. The beliefs which people hold about themselves and about the possibility of change, whether in a group context or some other, will have a significant bearing on their success. Second, is the motivation needed to prepare for a group and sustaining your groupwork; understanding what nourishes your motivation will help to maintain it. Third, it is important to be aware of your likely strengths in the group and what you might find difficult, or what might lie outside your 'comfort zone'.

> I find it difficult to handle indifferent feedback – preferring it to be positive or negative. I think this is because it makes it hard to know where I stand as a groupworker, as I am keen to adapt the group as feedback is received.
> Portfolio W, 5.1

Finally, a self-audit about what you like about groups will be illuminating. It will prompt you to take a step back to consider that your own preferences may not necessarily be shared by your co-workers or group members.

> As a group member, positive experiences of groups have been those where there is a clear outline of what will happen, so that significantly unexpected

events do not occur. This leads to a feeling of security and enables me to enjoy the group; for example, a 'learn to ski' group, where each session had a list of new skills that the participant would learn through the course of a lesson.

Portfolio S, 1.1

Understanding the group leadership

The group leadership is another system in the group; sometimes, when there are three or more co-workers this constitutes a group in itself. The personal qualities of the group leadership and the way in which you relate to one another and to the other systems in the group, is crucial to the way the group will be experienced. In particular, there needs to be a mutual understanding of the significance of *social location*, in terms of gender, race, sexuality, age, class, etc. in the co-leadership group, and also how this is likely to relate to the social location of group members. For the four white women who co-led the Memory Joggers group (Box 1.J), the main differences of significance were ones of professional status, as Jenny explains:

> As a 'group' of four it felt powerful when working and planning together. In a sense it gave strength to the [larger] group. However, a power difference was apparent within the four facilitators. I often felt that Jill and I were expected to take the lead or that, on occasions, we did anyway. Joy, in particular, felt that if Jill or I made a suggestion then it should stand simply because 'you're qualified and know more than us'.
>
> Portfolio J, 2.P&O

The group leadership needs to develop what is sometimes referred to as emotional literacy (Goleman, 1996). The problem in discussing feelings about status in the Memory Joggers' co-leadership were mirrored in an avoidance of focusing on feelings in the group itself.

> Where I think we lack experience as co-workers in ending sessions is failure to discuss 'feeling'. Activities are discussed, members are focused on what has been achieved and we highlight successes. Members say that they have enjoyed themselves and look forward to coming, and I believe these remarks to be genuine ... However, in summing up we have never mentioned anxiety levels rising as members feel challenged, or had lengthy discussion about how they feel as regards memory loss. Perhaps it's our fear of being rejected by members, and dealing explicitly with memory deficit is challenging.
>
> Portfolio J, 2.1

Co-working is considered in more detail in Chapter 6.

Understanding the group members[1]

There are three levels at which an understanding of the group members is important. The first belongs to a more general level, of group members as 'young offenders' or 'women with severe mental health problems':

The idea for this particular group arose in discussion between the co-workers who identified a number of common themes among several female clients with long-term severe mental health problems, namely:

- poor understanding of the nature of their mental illness
- lack of awareness of viable alternatives to coping with their problems
- low self-confidence and self-esteem resulting from their experiences of mental illness.

We were also aware that none of the women had experienced this type of groupwork before, and that many experienced social isolation, which we hoped to partially address through the group process.

Portfolio W, 2.1

The second level is an understanding of this group in particular. How does this group respond and how can it get the best out of itself? Orla demonstrates this in respect of the Offending Awareness group (Box 1.O).

As the term *role play* had caused concern in a previous session, the technique was 'marketed' under the heading of placing themselves 'in some-one else's Adidas'.

Portfolio O, 4.2

The third is at the level of the individual member, and an awareness of the particular strengths, potential and challenges of each person. Degrees of understanding will usually increase with contact, and groups are more likely to show individuals off in a variety of different lights, as Helen observes in respect of Hayley, a member of the Women of Hope group (Box 1.H):

Hayley was having a lot of support outside the group ... weekly therapy, local drop-in service, GP and psychiatric input. Despite this Hayley was always negative. Much of her conversation was around nobody cared ... Yet she had another side to her character, which manifested itself in the group – caring, good sense of humour, thoughtful and considerate.

Portfolio H, 5.1

Outer systems

Practitioners sometimes make the mistake of neglecting the outer systems, explored below, thinking them to be remote and exerting less pull. In fact, these outer systems can be by far the most powerful in the group, even determining whether the group will exist or not.

Understanding your team and agency

Jenny, a social worker in a Community Mental Health team, was disappointed and distressed to discover how the Memory Joggers group was perceived by some of the other professionals in the team.

To my dismay I have realised that not all colleagues are as supportive as I had once believed and that groupwork is seen *as a soft option*. This is incredible, as I find the project absolutely draining at times!

Portfolio J, 2.1

The success of groupwork in the longer term depends on team and agency support even though they might never have contact with an individual group (see Chapter 9). Team colleagues can sometimes actively oppose new developments (Rushton and Martyn, 1990). Despite the rhetoric of user-led services, there is more likely to be support for a group when it is presented as meeting the needs of the team or agency. This is acceptable as long as this is consistent with the needs of the group members. For example, in addition to helping young people leaving care, Samantha also identified that 'there is a need for the Leaving Care team to become better acquainted with young people other than those on their individual caseloads. The group will provide a good opportunity for this' (Portfolio S, 2.1). Whole-team involvement in the planning also meant that colleagues felt confident about inviting their 'own' young people.

BOX 2.3   GROUP CONTEXT

Westville Women's group

Wendy is a white social worker in Westville Community Mental Health team. Her co-worker, **Win**, is a social work assistant. (See Box 1.W.)

Wendy writes:

The team is multi-disciplinary and consists of three Community Psychiatric Nurses, two Social Workers, an Occupational Therapist, a Social Work Assistant, two Community Support Workers and a secretary. We work with people who suffer from severe and enduring mental health problems, typically schizophrenia, manic depression or long-term depression or anxiety problems.

Each team member holds a caseload of service users, which involves working with individuals, carers and families. Because most of the people whom the team works with have fairly complex needs, usually two or more team members are involved in working with each person and we try to make sure that all users are known to each team member. The team already runs a number of groups including a weekly social support group, a weekly activity based group, and a twice weekly gardening group. I am involved in helping to run all of these groups on a rota basis.

The co-leader for the proposed Women's group is Win, who is the social work assistant in the team. Win also holds her own caseload and is involved in the running of all of the above groups.

Portfolio W, 1.1

It is important that the whole team owns the work and puts the effort in, particularly practical support such as providing transport.

Portfolio S, 2.1

ACTIVITY 2.3: MAKING CONTACT WITH OUTER SYSTEMS

- Given the context for the proposed Women's group (Box 2.3), what team needs do you think the group might satisfy? (You may need to speculate by supplying your own additional information.) Make a list in a left-hand column.
- What potential objections can you foresee Wendy's team might raise? Make a list in a central column.
- What responses could you give to counter the potential objections you have identified? Make a list in a right-hand column.

Understanding significant others

Group members spend much more time outside the group than in it, even when the context is group care. The value and meaning of the group's time together should be set against the impact of families, communities, other professionals and the legal system on the group members. From the point of view of the group these may seem to be outer systems, but for many of the group members they are distinctly central. This is explored in greater detail in Chapter 8.

KEY POINTS

- Groupwork is underpinned by different kinds of knowledge derived from research, practitioners and group members themselves.
- Groupwork is also underpinned by knowledge from key disciplines such as philosophy, politics, social and organisational psychology.
- No single model of groupwork is able to take account of the great variety of groupwork methods and contexts.
- Each group has a unique 'fingerprint' composed of a different balance of the same basic seven elements.
- Systems theories help to understand how to work with groups and promote groupwork effectively.

FURTHER READING

AASWG (1999), *Standards for Social Work Practice with Groups,* Association for the Advancement of Social Work with Groups: www.aaswg.org

These provide a basic set of standards for knowledge, values and tasks as the 'distinguishing features of group work'.

Brown, A. (1994), *Groupwork* [3rd edition], Aldershot: Arena.

This is a classic text on groupwork and it remains highly relevant and readable.

Garvin, C.D., Gutiérrez, L.M. and Galinsky, M.J. (eds) (2004), *Handbook of Social Work with Groups*, New York: Guilford Press.

An encyclopaedic handbook, not to be read 'at one sitting', but with useful chapters covering the broad range of social work with groups.

Ward, D. (2002), 'Groupwork' in R. Adams, L. Dominelli and M. Payne (eds), *Social Work: themes, issues and critical debates* [2nd edition], Basingstoke: Macmillan.

A succinct, chapter-long account, looking at the challenges to groupwork as a mainstream practice.

FOOTNOTE

1   As an aside, I am drawn to the term 'group member'. It is an especially inclusive term, since it also embraces group leaders – they are members of the group too, albeit with a different role. It is hugely better than any of the various terms which describe the people who use social services – user, service user, client, customer, etc. Whatever the next incarnation of 'service user', group members will continue to be group members.

CHAPTER 3

PREPARE

OBJECTIVES

By the end of this chapter you will be able to:

▓ Make preparations for a new group or revitalise an existing group

▓ Understand different methods of deciding how group membership can be decided, and use these in an inclusive way

▓ Present the potential purposes of a group in a 'manifesto'

▓ Balance structure with flexibility in preparing individual group sessions

▓ Know how to debrief in order to prepare for future sessions.

PREPARING FOR A GROUP

Establishing a planning group

A key and recurring theme of this book is the need for groupworkers to think strategically when planning and preparing for a group, especially since the success of a group can be undermined by lack of support from colleagues. Moreover, for a successful group to become a successful groupwork service, the group leaders must attract wide support. You can begin to develop these alliances from the start by establishing a planning group and considering who should be part of this. The planning group should not be involved in the details of the group and it need not be bureaucratic – it may only need to meet once or twice – but it can play a significant role in identifying the necessary resources and legitimising the group. The planning group can help with matters such as publicity, and its support could be critical if there are difficult decisions to be made around staffing.

Once the group itself is established, the planning group can also be reconvened to receive reports of progress, so that the group's impact can be properly acknowledged. By cultivating the planning group's connection to the group itself, the groupworkers can strengthen agency support.

ACTIVITY 3.1: THE PLANNING GROUP

1   Which key people should be members of the planning group for your proposed group?
2   What tasks would the planning group have?
3   How will potential group members be included in the planning group?

If you are not yet at the stage of considering your own group, consider these three questions in respect of one of the groups in Box 3.1.
(An example response is given in the Appendix.)

Where agencies have already committed themselves to a groupwork programme it is likely to be an established 'package', such as Crimestop and Parents Plus in this book. In these cases, groupworkers have the advantage of pushing at an open door, though a planning group may still be appropriate to consider how this 'off-the-shelf' package might be customised to the particular context (see later).

Groupworkers might avoid establishing a planning group because of lack of time, or because they fear that their own ideas for the group will be swamped by others. Although there are always risks when opening up your ideas for a group to others, these are outweighed by the benefits described above.

As well as deepening support in the agency, a planning group can widen support in the community. Including people in the planning group who represent marginalised groups in the community, or can at least reach out to them, will help to ensure that people from minority groups are not excluded from membership of the group.

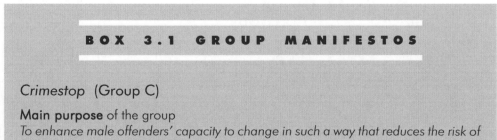

BOX 3.1 GROUP MANIFESTOS

Crimestop (Group C)

Main purpose of the group
To enhance male offenders' capacity to change in such a way that reduces the risk of their victimising other people.

Box 3.1 continued

Firwood Family Support group (Group F)

Main purpose of the group
To provide family support in the Firwood area, bringing families together for mutual support in a neutral and safe environment, reducing isolation and vulnerability. We aim to provide practical resources such as a toy library and a clothing exchange. Outside agencies will be invited to offer advice on issues such as health, benefits, children's behaviour.

Westville Women's group (Group W)

Main purpose of the group
a) *to offer a group experience for women who, because of their particular mental health needs, are typically not offered this type of approach of opportunity*
b) *to promote self-confidence and esteem*
c) *to promote greater understanding of mental health issues as relating to women.*

Purpose

In Chapter 2 we considered the importance of researching the need for a group. If this has been successful, the purposes of the group will flow from the need. It is vital to make a clear and succinct statement of the purpose, such as those in Box 3.1. These purposes are provisional, since they may change as you approach potential group members on an individual basis, but they provide the initial 'manifesto' for the group, and the basis for the planning group to decide on resources and support.

The purposes of the group will have an impact on the kind of preparations you need to make. The best way to consider how purposes influence preparation is to build a profile of the group's 'contours'. If you give careful consideration to each of the eleven contours in Box 3.2 you will be able to make preparations which are appropriate to your group and which avoid drifting into some kind of default group – a one and a half hour group for eight members meeting weekly for eight weeks. This default may well suit the purposes of your proposed group, but you need to check this, and the eleven contours will help.

A group for women who have experienced sexual abuse as children is likely to require considerable intimacy, suggesting a smaller membership with a greater degree of similarity between members and a relatively frequent meeting pattern; a group of tenants on a public housing estate would be likely to benefit from wide and diverse participation, perhaps meeting monthly rather than weekly to allow for task completion.

BOX 3.2   GROUP CONTOURS

1   **Group history**   *Established* ....*New*
Is this a revitalisation of an existing group? Will some or all people know each other, or will all group members be new to one another?

2   **Leadership**   *Self-help* ....*Practitioner-led*
To what extent will the group rely on professional leadership? Will leadership style change during the life of the group?

3   **Choice**   *Voluntary* ....*Compulsory*
Will all or any group members be required to join the group? For those who attend 'voluntarily' will there be any kinds of pressure to join?

4   **Group mix**   *Different* .... *Similar*
Will the group benefit from the intimacy of similar biographies and circumstances, or the variety and challenge arising from difference?

5   **Size**   *Large* .... *Small*
Should the group be relatively public and campaigning or relatively intimate and private? How many members are needed to make it viable?

6   **Extent**   *Open-ended* .... *Time-limited*
How long is it likely to take for the group to fulfil its purpose? What are the (dis)advantages of having an agreed end-point for the group?

7   **Joining–Leaving**   *Open* .... *Closed*
Should group members be able to join and leave at different times during the group's life? What are the practical realities?

8   **Session duration**   *Long* .... *Short*
How long are group members likely to be able to concentrate in the group? Will travel arrangements affect the duration of the sessions?

9   **Interval**   *Seldom*..*Frequent*
How often does the group need to meet to maintain its momentum and achieve its purposes? Will it meet at the same intervals throughout?

10   **Focus**   *Outward*.. *Inward*
To what extent will the content of group sessions focus on the group as a group, and to what extent on what happens outside the group?

11   **Structure**   *Loose* .... *Tight*
How 'scripted' will group sessions be and what room for extemporisation will there be? Is the degree of structure likely to change over time?

ACTIVITY 3.2: GROUP PURPOSE AND PREPARATION

Draw up a draft Group Manifesto for your proposed group, using the examples in Box 3.1 as a guide.

Consider each of the factors in the Group Contours (Box 3.2) and draw up a profile for your proposed group.

If you are not yet at the stage of considering your own group, take one of the groups in Box 3.1 and develop a Group Profile for it (you will need to refer to Chapter 1 for more details about each of these groups).

Revitalising an existing group

The Firwood Family Support group (Box 1.F) has been meeting for over a year. The families in the group have non-intensive social services involvement. Fran, one of the social workers, is concerned that the group needs revitalising.

> We are looking at trying to encourage more people to join our group – fresh blood – and one of the methods we are using is to design and print a flyer. We will then advertise in local libraries, health centres and attend meetings of health professionals in order to promote this resource. We feel this may act as preventative, pro-active social work instead of reactive.
>
> Portfolio F, 1.1

Preparing established groups for a new role including new members, requires a different approach to planning a group *de novo*. New members may well take their cue from existing members, with the result that the group changes only in size not in substance. In addition to inviting new members, a group wishing to revitalise should also re-consider its purposes and decide whether the group needs more fundamental changes – a different venue, new methods, even a new name?

Membership

Who will be members of the group? There are four ways in which people are likely to become group members:

1   *Self-selected* from an open pool of eligible people. Eligibility is often defined by a single criterion or specific community of interest (any individual who misuses alcohol; any resident of this apartment block; any person who has an interest in improving nursery provision in this area).

2   *Recruited* in a variety of ways, through publicity and referral by other professionals. Some potential groups members may already be in contact with professional services, but not all.

3   *Selected* by the group leaders as people who they consider are likely to benefit from the group. All group members are known to the group leaders or their colleagues.

4   *Required* to attend the group, perhaps to fulfil a legal obligation such as a Court
      Order. Compulsory membership is considered in more detail in Chapter 4.

Social action groups are characterised by category 1 membership (see *Groupwork*
Jjournal, 2004, 14.2 for a comprehensive introduction to social action groupwork).
Many of the groups in this category are running without the support or even the
knowledge of the professional services. Groups in Probation and Youth Offending Teams
are likely to have memberships in category 4, such as the Crimestop and Offending
Awareness groups. The other groups illustrating this book fall into categories 2 or 3,
and this reflects most of the groups in the Groupwork Project. The Family Support
group is the nearest to category 1.

Group membership is a central concern in the preparation stage and the way in
which people become members has an impact on the group itself. In all categories, the
question of who is eligible to join the group is central, and this should be clearly linked
to the group's purpose. Discussing purpose and eligibility with the team, or a wider
planning group, is not always straightforward, but it is likely to help groupworkers to
rehearse their reasons:

> When we discussed the idea for the group [for women with mental health
> problems] in the whole team, one male team member said that many of the
> men whom we worked with also suffered from low self-esteem, difficulties
> in assertiveness or communication.
>
> Portfolio W, 2.1

This challenge to Wendy about the needs of men in similar situations to the women for
her proposed group enabled her to make the case openly for an all-women's group,
whilst also logging the need for a men's group, too. Following open discussion and the
recording of the criteria, Wendy noted that 'there was no disagreement over group
membership once criteria were established' (Portfolio W, 2.1).

One of the key questions about membership is who has the power to decide
membership. Being *in-group* or *out-group* can arouse memories from the school yard of
being picked (or not) to join a team or gang. In those situations where the workers offer
the group as a service, there is a responsibility to ensure that the group composition is
appropriate to purpose and sometimes this will mean saying no. An individual's behaviour
or circumstances may be so different from others that there is real concern that the
group may not be able to function, or that individuals in the group (including the
person in question) may be put at emotional or physical risk.

Relying on others to make these judgements also carries risks, as Mandy found in
relation to the Managing Behaviour group (Box 1.M):

> Mavis [the Homefinder] was our link person and when we approached her
> about this group she was very interested, yet, I didn't feel we had any control
> of the selection of the group members. Mavis chose the people *she* felt were
> in need of this group, and many of the guidelines we had asked her to use
> had (unintentionally) been ignored.
>
> Portfolio M, 1.P&O

ACTIVITY 3.3: EXCLUSION AND INCLUSION

Take the draft Group Manifesto which you developed in Activity 3.2 (or one of the examples in Box 3.2 if you are not yet in a position to consider your own group). What criteria will you use to decide who should be eligible for membership of the group? Who would you exclude from the group? How would you justify this? How would you enforce it?

We will consider ways to prepare individuals for group membership in the next chapter.

Practicalities

The success of any one group is highly dependent on mundane but very time-consuming practicalities. There were many factors which propelled 54 of the 68 (79%) groups in the Groupwork Project to a successful launch (Box 1.1), but it became clear during consultations that practical problems loomed large for the one in five groups which failed to fly. Here is a checklist of significant factors.

√ Funding

What basic resources will the group require in order to function well? The group might generate these funds for itself through its activities or it may be possible to apply for start-up grants. There are advantages in working together to produce funds and then spending these in a tangible way; however, the group does not want to be oppressed by the need for constant work on activities which might not have any other value. Clearly, this should be a discussion which the group has with itself.

Wendy wanted to plan for two possible activity days for the Women's group (see Box 3.3):

> I applied to Social Services and got a small grant of £30. I also applied to Health Promotion and we received funding of £100. This was needed to subsidise two activity days which we hoped to offer, to pay for any equipment and handouts and to pay for things like refreshments.
>
> Portfolio W, 2.1

In the Memory Joggers group, Jenny and her co-workers understood the importance of securing their manager's understanding of the needs of the group, which resulted in practical support:

> Javid [the team manager] was supportive and secured us the sum of money we requested to purchase items for the group. He also set aside £100 for useful texts to be used not only for the purpose of the group but also for the whole Community Mental Health Team. Javid knew we were committed and he, too, saw the long-term benefits for service users and because of this he offered his full support.
>
> Portfolio J, 2.1

The preparations for the group include decisions about what will be appropriate to expect group members to supply and what should be provided. These should be provisional decisions which can usually be revisited once the group meets and begins to find its voice.

√ Time / Timing

It has always interested me that 'lack of time' is such a common reason given for not working with groups. What this really means is 'lack of priority', perhaps linked to the fact that groupwork is relatively high profile. The semi-public nature of groupwork means that the consequences of poor preparation and short-cuts are much more visible than work with individuals. The need for time to prepare and work with groups is self-evident, but what can be overlooked is the practical problem of *timing*. I have experienced this with two groups, both well-advanced in preparation, but where a time could not be found which suited enough of the people involved.

Compromises and choices will invariably have to be made around times and timings. Paul reflects on the possible consequences for the Parents Plus group of the need to accommodate his holiday plans:

> One concession revolved around my annual leave arrangements: our group would meet for three consecutive weekly sessions, break for two weeks then meet again on five consecutive weekly occasions. While one session would have had to be missed anyway as this was the Bank Holiday, I did wonder whether meeting my particular needs would involve too long a break for the group.
>
> Portfolio P, 2.1

Paul's co-worker, Petra, also 'wondered if running the group on Monday mornings put some members off' (Portfolio P1, 3.1).

The timing for Orla and her colleagues was especially problematic since many of the young offenders would be engaged in education or employment (or searching for employment) and were also subject to curfews for the first three months of their sentence, often from as early as 7:00pm. Groups had, therefore, to run from 4:00 to 6:00pm as the only time unaccounted for, though those in full-time employment might still find this problematic.

√ Venue and access

> The Centre was chosen as a venue for the group sessions as the building is not formal. It is away from the Social Services offices and is accessible to anyone who is disabled; this would hopefully enable the group members to feel at ease in this environment.
>
> Portfolio F, 2.1

Like moving to a new home, choosing the venue is usually a trade-off. Finding a place which is accessible to all group members, which has the necessary facilities such as a kitchen and cupboards to lock the group's belongings away between sessions, which is comfortable and which does not break the budget is unlikely. One or other of these desirables will doubtless have to be sacrificed.

Some teams have access to a room which is dedicated to groupwork. This is another advantage of broadening support for groupwork so that it can be seen as a regular part of professional practice and the agency's services. However, there are times when the group might wish to be physically separate from the agency and meet in a more neutral, community venue. Group members will appreciate a venue which fits well with the rest of their lives:

> The location of the [group] venue adjacent to the local bus station and town centre shops allowed for the possibility for group members of using time either side of the group for different things.
>
> Portfolio P, 2.1

√ Transport

For many groups transport can be the single most important factor. My first experience of groupwork was in rural East Anglia as an unqualified social worker, where I spent more time arranging and providing transport than in the groups themselves. However, this was essential work to bring isolated people together.

Public transport is a metaphor for groupwork, bringing people together for similar journeys, sharing the same vehicle to get from one place to another. It is a vital social service, keeping families and communities together – or not. Good public transportation has an enormous impact on the social fabric, and groupwork can prosper much more easily in these contexts. However, costly but uncosted professional time often plugs the gap of an inadequate transport system.

> We [the planning group] discussed the offer of the mini-bus, but agreed that we needed something more reliable (we may not have use of the mini-bus every week). We all agreed that staff would transport service users. Transport is an important issue. Many services run into problems because of the lack of transport provision, especially services for older people who are more reluctant either because they can't manage public transport or require door-to-door service.
>
> Portfolio J, 2.1

What is a necessity can also be an opportunity:

> It was an advantage that we were transporting members. It gave us the opportunity to reassure and relax people on arrival at the first session.
>
> Portfolio J, 3.2

√ Health and safety

When we gather people together we have a responsibility for their care and you should consider the particular needs of the people in the group to make appropriate preparations. There should be access to a First Aid box and fire hazards need to be considered along with access, especially for disabled people and any persons using a wheelchair. You are not necessarily the best qualified person to complete a risk assessment, but you do have an obligation to make sure others have.

In Box 3.3 you can see how Wendy addressed some of these practicalities in preparing for the Westville Women's group.

BOX 3.3 PRACTICALITIES

Westville Women's roup

We decided, after consulting the literature and thinking about the type of group we wanted, to aim for between 6 and 8 group members. This felt small enough for members to feel comfortable, and large enough to be able to do activities. We had a number of women in mind who fitted the criteria. We asked the team for referrals.

Practical details included:

Choice of venue. Due to financial limitations we decided to opt for Westville Health Centre, where we work, which is free. It has appropriate facilities, i.e. a large room which can be made private, an attached kitchen, toilet, etc. It is a non-smoking building so breaks need to be included. It is also not conveniently situated for everyone we have in mind, so transport in our own cars needs to be provided. I think transport was important in terms of attendance. When transport hasn't been provided for other groups run by the team, attendance has dropped.

Funding was also a planning issue. I applied to Social Services and got a small grant of £30. I also applied to Health Promotion, and we received funding of £100. Funding was needed to subsidise two activity days which we hoped to offer; to pay for any equipment and handouts we hoped to give to group members; and to pay for things like refreshments.

Contacts needed to be made in the planning stage to gain access to potential resources and request speakers. For example, contact was made with Shire Well

> **Box 3.3 continued**
>
> Women's Centre and with the local Police Community Liaison Office for help with organising sessions on women and health, and women and safety.
>
> **Resources** also needed to be gathered. For example, we gathered material from the Health Promotion Resource Centre and from Shire Library before planning the sessions.
>
> **A time** for the group had to be arranged. We made a list of times when both ourselves and the room were available, and decided to put this to potential group members for negotiation.
>
> Portfolio W, 2.1

'Off-the-shelf' programmes

Some groupworkers find themselves delivering an 'off-the-shelf' group to a manual's specification. The advantages of having a ready-tested format has to be balanced against the possibility of having to squeeze *this* group into *that* manual. Two of the illustrative groups, Crimestop and Parents Plus (Boxes 1.C and 1.P), were ready-programmed. Paul, co-leader of the latter, had a clear understanding that his involvement with a training programme in general groupwork would help him to make the group programme work for the group, rather than the group working for the programme (Portfolio P, 2.1; Sharry and Fitzpatrick, 2001). Claire, co-leader of Crimestop, also came to understand that the planning task was rather different when a group runs to a manual.

> Planning for this group was less about creating content, as this was already laid down in a manual. Planning for me was centred on the co-working relationship and on applying the material to a particular group.
>
> Portfolio C, 2.1

PREPARING FOR INDIVIDUAL SESSIONS

> Sessions that have been focused have worked extremely well, giving a spontaneous reaction, in comparison to sessions that have had no set focus or agenda.
>
> Portfolio F, 2.1

How much preparation?

Fran's paradox (above), that spontaneity is released rather than inhibited by structure, reflects a dilemma which exercises all groupworkers – how much preparation? A stock answer suggests that this should relate to the group's purpose, ranging from most structure for groups in the social control and educational categories to some structure for social action and social support, and little structure for therapeutic (see Chapter 2). However, it is not so much the degree of structure as its flexibility that is important. All groups benefit from preparation, and almost all of these are helped by a programme of sorts. The extent to which groupworkers are able to improvise when necessary is of more consequence than the degree of structure *per se*. Inexperienced groupworkers are likely to stick hard and fast or drift aimlessly in roughly equal measure.

Constructing (and deconstructing) a session

Groupworkers in the Groupwork Project (Box 1.1) found it helpful to prepare a 'play-list' for each session, similar to that in Box 3.4. The discussion which culminates in the final version of the play-list is likely to lead to a more thoughtful session, especially if the group as a whole can play its part in the process. This is not always possible or appropriate, certainly early in a group's life, but it is something to which the group should aspire.

The play-list acts as a cribsheet to remind groupworkers of the nature and order of the activities that have been planned. The sequence of activities may be particularly important, perhaps linked to desired changes in mood and tempo during the session. Lengthy discussions may have been necessary to arrive at some agreement about this, so the final play-list is an important reminder of what has been decided. The co-workers may also want to put an initial by each element to remind them who will be taking the lead, with approximate timings. A side-note of the necessary equipment and materials (the group's 'props') is also useful.

I should emphasise that preparing for a session, even to the extent of drawing up a play-list, does not mean that every minute must somehow be filled. When we look carefully at Helen's play-list for the Women of Hope group (Box 3.4), it is apparent that the bulk of the session (particularly items 3 to 6) is open to whatever the group members choose to introduce into the session. What Helen and her co-worker have done is to provide prompts and structures which they hope will encourage the members to feel able to make best use of the group's time. Much of their groupworking skill will rely on their ability to respond to what happens in the group in this unfilled time.

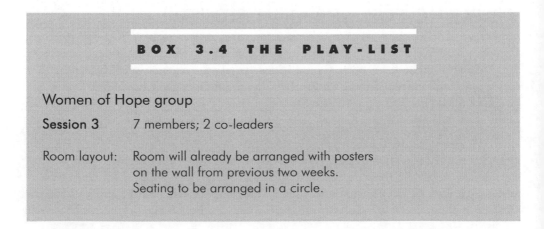

BOX 3.4 THE PLAY-LIST

Women of Hope group

Session 3   7 members; 2 co-leaders

Room layout: Room will already be arranged with posters
on the wall from previous two weeks.
Seating to be arranged in a circle.

Box 3.4 continued   *PROPS:*

Small table in the middle with booklet on anxiety and other information on depression, signs and symptoms, etc. Refreshments on a table at the back of the room. Music to be played very quietly in the background.	*Information booklets* *Tape*

Group name: 'Women of Hope' on a flipchart board; this is a decorative poster.   *Women of Hope flipchart sheet*

Opening statement:

1   Welcome group members – thank them for coming, run through session format and check this is OK.

Warm-up: *

2   Spend a few minutes at the beginning doing an exercise to help people relax and communicate with each other.   *Set of 18 cards with an item on each*

Items in this session:

3   After the warm-up, we will spend time hearing from anyone who would care to share with the group – how things were for them during the last week or any issues they wish to bring to the group.

4   We would also like to have feedback on the group so far.

5   We will then break for refreshments.   *Tea, coffee,*

6   In the second half of the session we will focus on any issues that we need to address from the first part of the session.   *milk, sugar, biscuits. Prompt for relaxation*

7   We will finish with a relaxation exercise and a reading called The Beach'.   *exercise; copy of 'The Beach'*

* **Warm-up:**   **Links**

Each member, including the leaders, will be given two cards [from a pre-written set]. In turn we will read out each card, and place ourselves on an imaginary diagonal line across the room, depending on whether we really like, really dislike or are indifferent to whatever is written on the card (e.g. hot curries).

Adapted from Portfolio H, 4.1

ACTIVITY 3.4: PREPARING THE PLAY-LIST

Women of Hope group
As a co-leader in the Women of Hope group, your experience of Session 3 is that the women were very unforthcoming during item 3 (see Box 3.4), and this affected the rest of the group session.

What reasons might explain the group members' reticence? How would these reasons affect your preparations for the next session?

Draw up a play-list for the next meeting (Session 4, meeting one week later) based on your analysis of why Session 3 did not work well.

Each session of the group needs constructing with flexibility in mind. In the Offending Awareness group, Orla demonstrated how effective groupwork usually relies on varying the degree of structure within one session quite deliberately to achieve different effects.

> The session was structured quite tightly during the first activity; had the young people not understood fully the purpose and structure of the first activity, they may have experienced great difficulties completing the second activity which was more loosely structured. This involved preparing dialogue then filming their role plays. This approach allowed the group members to express themselves more freely and develop skills they often have no opportunity to use, such as decision-making and prioritizing the content of their 'scripts'. This lesser degree of structure allowed group members to take ownership of the activity as a project of their own creation. A direct result of this was that the group became more cohesive, worked together, and behaved well throughout, despite the potential for disorder of this looser structure.
>
> Portfolio O, 4.1

In the Memory Joggers group, Jenny and her co-facilitators learned that the group responded to a very structured first half, with a slightly less structured second half. 'Group members became stressed if left to make their own decisions and often struggled to move things forward throughout the memory section. They also tended to be more comfortable with limited choice in the second half' (Portfolio J, 4.1). Preparation for group sessions is most successful when it is based on the accumulating experience of how this particular group responds.

Preparing the physical environment

The physical environment has a substantial impact on the group (Phillips, 2001). I described earlier the impossibility of finding the ideal venue for a group, but it is possible to mitigate some of the disadvantages of the site for the group by preparing the physical environment, as Wendy notes below.

We found we needed to spend time planning the physical environment. As the group met in a Health Centre, the environment wasn't immediately suitable, and we needed to adapt it to make it feel comfortable and welcoming.

Portfolio W, 2.1

The shape of the group is important. To facilitate good all-round eye and other non-verbal contact a circle or horse-shoe of chairs is often preferred. The groupworkers need to decide whether they will shape the group's space before members arrive (if they have the opportunity) or whether group members should be involved in this. Where will co-workers sit in relation to each other (side by side, at 'six o'clock', 'eight o'clock', etc. to each other)? What kinds of equipment and props will be required, and can these be tested out beforehand? In preparing for the group's fourth or fifth session, for example, do the groupworkers want to shape the meeting space differently in order to trigger some changes in the group? What opportunities for physical changes are there during any single session?

Though it is difficult to cite hard evidence, I believe that shaping the space which the group will occupy is a significant factor in the group's success. It is usually quite appropriate for groupworkers to use their expertise and to be 'good hosts' for the group. Orla describes a situation which is as near to the perfect venue as a groupworker could ask for, but not everyone is so fortunate:

We were extremely lucky in being provided with new premises specifically for the clients of our programme, and thus we could furnish and organise the rooms in a way which we felt would facilitate a relaxed atmosphere and show the young people that they were worthy of a calm and well-maintained area in which to work ... the building itself is located centrally in the town in an area familiar to the young people due to its proximity to many of the solicitors' firms they may have had contact with via their involvement with the criminal justice system.

Portfolio O, 2.1

Prepare for the unexpected

Preparing for a group is as much a psychological process as a physical one. Thinking through potential obstacles to the success of any particular session gives you the opportunity to rehearse alternative strategies to overcome them. Though the unexpected can never be banished, it can be reduced by imaginative discussion prior to the session, and it can be useful to share any bad fantasies with your co-workers, and to listen to theirs. You need to hold on to the fact that these *are* fantasies and highly improbable! This is all part of the tuning-in process, a well-established routine for groupworkers to prepare themselves for working with a group (Shulman, 1999).

It is always useful to have a Plan B, especially for those parts of a group session where you can reasonably predict a problem, and especially if you are relying on outsiders to join the group. Wendy describes the difficulties encountered when the programme relied on a guest. She also points to the learning curve which enabled preparation to become more meaningful from one session to another:

On two occasions, guest speakers pulled out at short notice and we had to take over the sessions ourselves ... we prepared on a weekly basis as we became more aware of the types of activity which the women responded to best.

Portfolio W, 2.1

It is hard to know how to be prepared for what faced Jenny for the first meeting of the Memory Joggers group: the venue had been vandalised. Nevertheless, she and her co-workers restored the rooms to some kind of order so that the session could go ahead. Ultimately, following persistent vandalism, the group moved to another venue, with consequent pluses and minuses for the group.

Positive – a permanent room for the group's use allowing us to become more established; nicer surroundings, brighter room, better facilities.
Negative – long corridors making transporting more problematic.

Portfolio J, 1.2

Each session is likely to provide at least one surprise and we can often learn the most from these unexpected events. Claire describes one such occurrence in the Crimestop group for adult offenders:

I was not prepared for one member's anger to be expressed in the form of complete silence – Ceiran did not speak until the team-building work was well underway, so when the anger was expressed verbally it was a shock.

Portfolio C, 3.2

Completing the loop

Preparation for one session relies on adequate reflection on the previous one. Claire experienced Ceiran's silence and subsequent outburst as a shock and was, therefore, perhaps unable to work with it in the way that she would have liked. It is vital that she is able to reflect on this, either immediately in the group, or more likely after the group with her co-worker or supervisor. We associate preparation with actions before an event, but preparation is in fact based on previous experiences and we only make best use of these if time is set aside to reflect on them. What is sometimes called debriefing is, therefore, also preparation for the next session.

This same process is just as important for the group as it is for the worker and the individual members. The beginning of one session of the group must connect with the ending of the previous session; and the ending of one session must anticipate the beginning of the next (there are particular issues to consider if the group consists of just one session, Ebenstein, 1999). This preparation might take the form of mental or physical tasks between one session or another, or it may be a form of 'check in' where members are asked to think about what they would like the group to take up when it next meets, and to comment briefly on their memories and feelings about the group from the previous session.

KEY POINTS

■ A small Planning Group is a key way in which others who are not directly involved in the groupwork can invest time and interest in the group.

■ There are four different ways in which group membership might be decided: self-selected, recruited, selected, required.

■ Group purpose will help determine the shape of the group, and this shape is composed of at least eleven 'contours'.

■ The practicalities are probably the most significant factors in the group's success, including the physical environment for the group.

■ Most groups benefit from structure, but only when this can be used flexibly; paradoxically, it is important to plan unplanned time.

FURTHER READING

Phillips, J. (2001) *Groupwork in Social Care: Planning and Setting up Groups*, London: Jessica Kingsley.

This book focuses especially on the preparation for groups in social work and social care and uses eight groups as illustrative case studies.

Sharry, J. (2001) *Solution-Focused Groupwork*, London: Sage.

Although this book goes well beyond the preparation stage of groupwork, it will provide you with an excellent guide to solution-focused groupwork as a practice method.

CHAPTER 4

MEET

OBJECTIVES

By the end of this chapter you should be able to:

▨ Plan how best to meet potential group members individually to offer the group

▨ Tune in to your own feelings and the possible feelings of group members

▨ Understand the impact of choice and compulsion on group processes

▨ Differentiate between outcomes, feelings, processes and contexts

▨ Negotiate ground rules together with group members

▨ Make connections between groups and teams.

For all the preparation, evaluation, recording and other important support structures for successful groupwork, a group is marked and remembered by its *meeting*. Like the notion of a team, a group is a nebulous term until it is given expression in its joining together. At that point the idea of a group becomes a reality.

MEETING POTENTIAL GROUP MEMBERS

A term as supposedly clear as 'meet' is, nevertheless, fuzzy. For example, the implication of people together in the same room is misleading. Meetings of minds are possible across great distances and, more likely in the twenty-first century, electronically. Traditional definitions of groupwork are challenged by those groups, such as internet ones, whose meeting can be effective even though not face to face (Meier, 2004; Smokowski *et al.,* 2001).

For some groups there is no new gathering, since the people involved already meet in some form and, even for those groups which are created, the meeting process often begins well in advance of the first session of the actual group.

Meeting beforehand

The significance of groupworkers arranging to meet with potential group members on an individual basis became apparent during the Groupwork Project (see Box 1.1). groupworkers' confidence was enhanced and group members valued the individual offer of groupwork. For groups whose membership will be recruited, selected or required to join (see Chapter 3), an individual offer can be critical. However, making appointments with people to discuss the idea of the group may be a relatively new experience, for worker and service user alike. For Wendy, writing to potential members of the Women's Group (Box 1.W), this was a revelation.

> All potential members were very excited at having received an appointment letter from us, and it made me realise how generally service users have little control over their contact with mental health workers.
>
> Portfolio W, 3.1

It is important to consider issues of language and literacy, but where appropriate, information about the group sent with the introductory letter means that potential members can prepare questions. In their preparations for the Parents Plus group (Box 1.P), Paul and Petra sent written information about the group in advance of their visit.

> There seems to be a clear case for forwarding literature to potential group members prior to an initial visit. This creates some degree of informal choice about whether or not, in the first place, a visit is allowed to proceed. During visits where leaflets had been forwarded, on a couple of occasions these were to hand and clearly had been read.
>
> Portfolio P, 3.1

Paul thought that the notion of 'a group' may be quite novel, so he used the individual meetings as an opportunity 'to reflect with potential members about any previous experiences of groups (including family, friends, employment, pastimes) to help them think about what would enable joining [the group] to be smoother' (Portfolio P, 3.1). Since these individual meetings are a rehearsal for the group itself, a visit at about the time of day and day of the week that the group is expected to run is a good idea where practical. Of course, these individual meetings are time-consuming, especially when co-workers make them jointly and sometimes it is possible to be opportunistic, as Mandy notes in respect of recruitment to the Managing Behaviour for Carers group (Box 1.M):

> Due to the time factor we found ourselves in a position where we were unable to visit three prospective members in their homes. Fortunately there was a training day for foster carers at the Family Centre the day before our group was to start, so it was arranged to speak to these carers individually during their lunch break. We found this situation less than ideal. However,

because of this arrangement we were approached directly by another carer who wished to join the group.

Portfolio M, 2.1

Personalised offers of groupwork can alert groupworkers to potential stresses in the group itself, though these must always be tentative and not self-fulfilling. Novice groupworkers might view these as problems or challenges to their own control, as Mandy noted when visiting possible members for the Managing Behaviour for Carers group:

> A few of the more experienced carers came over as being more confident and sure of themselves, this left me wondering if they were going to be a problem in the group, i.e. monopolising the group or being unwilling to take advice.

Portfolio M, 2.2

Orla was pleased to have foreknowledge of a particular characteristic of Omar, who joined the Offending Awareness group (Box 1.O):

> Omar seems to permanently grin, which can be unnerving for both staff and young people upon first meeting, particularly when discussing sensitive and serious issues!

Portfolio O, 1.3

The pre-meeting meant that Orla was alerted to Omar's inappropriate grinning, and she was able to mediate the group's response to this because she could anticipate its effect.

As well as an opportunity for you to share your draft 'manifesto' for the group (see Chapter 3), this is also a time for potential group members to let you know about their ideas for the group, to ask you questions in a private setting as opposed to the semi-public venue of the group, and to express any concerns. Sometimes these can be very unexpected, as Mandy noted:

> We asked Moira if she had any questions she would like to ask us. She said, 'Will there be a test at the end?'

Portfolio M, 1

Moira's reference to a potential obstacle to joining the group which Mandy would never have thought about was very useful, since Mandy was then able to reassure other potential members that there would not be any test, if this was one of their concerns.

ACTIVITY 4.1: CONCERNS OF POTENTIAL GROUP MEMBERS

What kinds of concerns are people likely to have about joining a proposed group? If you are planning your own group, what specific concerns might people have when you meet them to make the offer of groupwork?

Potential members may have concerns about how much they will be expected to disclose in a group, or the impact of differences between them and other group members.

> One of our potential clients was a gay man. We made it clear to him he was welcome to bring his partner to the group if he wished. He stated he did not always tell people his sexuality. We assured him that it was his choice as to what information he shared in the group ... He did not attend due to a family member's illness.
>
> Portfolio X, 2.P&O

Potential group members are assessing you as much as you are assessing them, listening to the tone of your voice, judging whether you are the kind of person they can trust, wondering what you and the group will be like. If you already know the person with whom you are discussing the group, you have the opportunity to customise your 'pitch'; Orla, for example, approached the group differently with different potential members. Even though they all faced the same prospect of a custodial sentence if they did not comply, this did not prevent an individually tailored offer. One person was known to be very outgoing and so Orla emphasised the fun aspect of the group, another was very direct in his manner so Orla was straightforward and matter of fact about the group. Another, Oscar, was anxious and rather worried by the prospect of the group, so Orla responded in yet another way:

> Oscar was very quiet and quite nervous and seemed genuinely disconcerted by the notion of groupwork. We discussed his fears about joining the group, which it seemed stemmed from the feeling that he would be the 'new boy' and would not know anyone in a group that was already formed. I stressed how he would be starting the group for the first time with others as the programme was new, but that there shouldn't be much chance for this kind of 'new boy' attitude to develop in the group as young people may join every other week regularly.
>
> Portfolio O, 3.1

Subsequent feedback from Oscar suggested that Orla's approach was successful. Some might describe it as 'spin', but Orla never described anything other than the reality of the group, but she chose to emphasise different facets of the group in order to respond to different concerns and attractions. On reflection, Orla wondered whether she provided enough detail of what would happen in the group sessions:

> With hindsight I feel that some people may have felt that groupwork would be a repetitive experience for them as they had already covered work in many of the areas I outlined on an individual basis. In reality, the group sessions covered much new work; as facilitators we had taken great care to introduce fresh activities to ensure the group provided new insight into issues. In future I would provide a little more detail as to work to be covered in order to allay fears of going over old ground for group members.
>
> Portfolio O, 3.1

ACTIVITY 4.2: MEETINGS WITH POTENTIAL GROUP MEMBERS

First, read the outline of the Managing Behaviour for Carers Group in Box 1.M on page 15. In particular, consider the three pen pictures of Marcia, Moira and Molly.

- Make a note of the factors that you would take into consideration for each of the three separate meetings with Marcia, Moira and Molly.
- Rehearse your offer of groupwork with each of them.

When you are in a position to meet potential group members for the group that you are planning, repeat this process in preparation for these meetings.

There may be occasions when it is appropriate for potential members to be invited to an offer of groupwork *as a group*. Samantha reflected in her portfolio how she would plan for the next Sound Start group (Box 1.S) for young people moving to independent accommodation:

> Next time I would organise a social event which all potential members could attend and enjoy a relaxed meeting. There would be opportunities to ask questions without feeling outnumbered and inhibited by the workers. As it will be a rolling programme, it would be good for previous members to come and give some feedback about their experience [from past Sound Start groups].
>
> Portfolio S, 3.1

Ironically, an agency where groupwork is institutionalised may offer less opportunity for a particular groupworker to play a full part in every aspect of the groupwork. Claire, a Probation Officer, writes:

> I would not often have the opportunity of offering this group to potential members. That is the task of the Court and Assessment team … They are unlikely to be trained [as a Crimestop groupworker] and in some cases are not up to date on groupwork provision. Hence some unsuitable referrals are made.
>
> Portfolio C, 3.1

Claire goes on to advocate assessment of all potential members by the groupworkers themselves, with a holding group for people before they join the main group to help with the timing of people joining a new run of Crimestop.

Choice

With the growth of groupwork in probation and youth offending services, it is often suggested that the social control elements of groupwork are becoming paramount (Yates, 2004). Groupwork with 'involuntary clients' is without doubt a significant sector (Rooney and Chovanec, 2004). Two of the examples in this book, the Crimestop and Offending

Awareness groups, had members who faced breach proceedings if they did not attend, triggering a return to court and a possible custodial sentence.

In some respects the situation is more straightforward in groups where members are mandated to join – the constraints on their choice are obvious and explicit. However, all groupworkers should bear in mind the ambivalence that is commonly felt about group membership. With the exception of some social action groups, membership of a group usually signifies there are problems, challenges and difficulties which have brought the person to the group (Staples, 2004). The act of joining the group is often the first significant step towards recognition of this difficulty, but most people have not 'chosen' to be in that situation. These implicit constraints on members' choice can make more demands of the groupworker's skills than the obvious resistance in a group of involuntary members.

Even when a group is nominally voluntary, it is important to remember the kinds of unseen pressures which there may be on people to join. Those who see themselves as needing and benefiting from the group are, nevertheless, likely to wish they were not in that situation.

> I doubted whether Pauline herself experienced what we would recognise as an unconditional choice about whether to attend or not. Her younger two daughters were named on the Child Protection Register, so that her own attitude, her willingness to co-operate would be subject to scrutiny and assessment.
>
> Portfolio P, 3.2

Jenny also recognised these unseen pressures when recruiting for the Memory Joggers group (Box 1.J):

> To what extent the group members' choice was totally voluntary is questionable. Many members may be wanting to please family members or us, the group facilitators.
>
> Portfolio J, 1.2

Potential group members should always be left in no doubt about the consequences of a refusal of the groupwork service; in most cases, this means ensuring they know that it does not compromise access to other services.

> Emphasis was given in the letter to the fact that Pat's son's place on the waiting list [for Children and Adolescents Mental Health Service] would in no way be jeopardised by accepting or declining the groupwork offer.
>
> Portfolio P, 3.1

In the case of the Sound Start group for young people about to move into independent living, Samantha's team 'decided that all young people who are registered with the [leaving care] project at 16 years old would be expected to attend the group' (Portfolio S, 2.1). Registration therefore carried obligations, and one of these was group involvement.

Later in this chapter we will consider the process of establishing ground rules as an important tool to expose issues of compulsion and choice, not just in membership of the group but in life more generally.

Do we know each other?

The dynamics of the group will be affected by the kinds of meetings which group members have outside the group. Claire, for example, was surprised by the connections amongst the Crimestop group members:

> I was not prepared for the amount of knowledge this particular group had about each other from outside … this made for a lot of solidarity and a reluctance for some people to go against the dominant thoughts or feelings of another.
>
> Portfolio C, 3.2

The challenge for the groupworker is how to ensure that it is the new behaviours and roles in the group that are reinforced by the contacts between group members outside the group, and not the behaviours which have been established outside the group that continue to be reinforced within it. This is a difficult call and I will suggest some practical ways of achieving success in the next chapter.

As well as knowledge of one another, any history which group members have with you or your co-workers will have an impact on the group, too. Samantha recognised that 'the way I offered groupwork to my "own" young people and to those I had not met before was quite different' (Portfolio S, 3.1). Once in the group itself you will need to emphasise regularly the difference in your role, making sparse reference to special knowledge you may have of a group member and, if needs be, talking with the individual outside the group to explain your new role. Other group members can become very resentful if the group leader's relationship with some members of the group is privileged.

Usually it helps to share your dilemma with the group: 'I have been open with the group from the very first session about the fact that I know Sean from our individual work together, and I have always tried to be fair and balanced about this, though I know that sometimes it can be difficult for us all – Sean, the rest of the group and me – to find that balance.' This kind of statement is likely to prompt a reasonable response because it is open and honest and it brings everyone together into the same boat – 'it can be difficult for us all' – and not just a case of the group leader trying to explain or justify him- or herself.

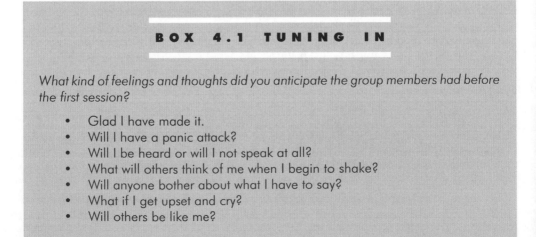

BOX 4.1   TUNING IN

What kind of feelings and thoughts did you anticipate the group members had before the first session?

- Glad I have made it.
- Will I have a panic attack?
- Will I be heard or will I not speak at all?
- What will others think of me when I begin to shake?
- Will anyone bother about what I have to say?
- What if I get upset and cry?
- Will others be like me?

Anticipating

All of the nine groupworkers whose groups illustrate this book wrote about the range of anticipatory feelings and thoughts which group members might have as they approach the first meeting of the group. Can you tell from the list in Box 4.1 which group this might be?[1] The fact that it is difficult to decide underlines the commonality of group processes, including the tuning-in technique. For Jenny, working with the Memory Joggers group, it was quite a revelation:

> Because I was so very positive about the whole project, it never seriously crossed my mind to consider the impact on the group members, their family and carers and how this might influence the session. I assumed they would think it was just wonderful.
>
> Portfolio J, 2.1

Wendy, running a similar group to Helen's, was clear that making time to tune in to their *own* feelings as co-workers, not just those of the group members, was critical to the success of the group:

> We found it especially useful as co-workers to discuss how we were feeling before each group. Usually we had similar feelings. For example, before a couple of sessions we both felt we'd have preferred not to go ahead with the group that day due to other pressing work commitments. This discussion broke the power of the feeling, and meant that we were able to put aside the other commitments and focus on the group. It also meant a shared understanding. We felt that if we had not done this, our unspoken feelings may have seeped into the group and [we may have] appeared distanced or flustered.
>
> Portfolio W, 3.2

Samantha had to confront the fact that her anticipatory feelings were coloured by the experience of failure to launch the Sound Start group on two previous occasions, each time with only one person turning up:

> Whilst waiting for group members to arrive, colleagues were teasing Sonia [my co-worker] and me about the other failed attempts and what had we done to turn them all away. I had to laugh at how difficult it had been to get just six people together to form a group. It was probably a rather hysterical way of addressing the silent fear that nobody would arrive again!
>
> Portfolio S, 3.2

MEETING FOR THE FIRST TIME

Despite all the preparations and the individual meetings before the first session of the group, it is always difficult to know what the chemistry of the individuals coming together will be and the difference *being in a group* makes.

Cards on the table

If you have called the group into being, it is natural that the group should look to you for leadership. We consider leadership issues in more detail in Chapter 6, but for now we will consider your responsibilities at the beginning of the group. At this time, the group looks to you and your co-worker to make an introduction. Though this need not be formal, it should amount to a clear statement of purpose, however expressed. Putting your cards on the table in this way helps group members to understand why you feel the group is worthwhile; this may in essence be a re-statement of the individual offer of groupwork, but it is symbolically important to make it to everyone at the same time.

The purpose of the group is usually more complex than a linear 'now we are here and we aim to be there then' approach. Of course, desired outcomes are important, but the group is most likely to have other kinds of purpose, too. These will be concerned with feelings and emotions (often referred to as the 'group affect'), the ways in which the group will develop to achieve its purposes (the group dynamics or group process) and the relationship of the group to the world outside the group (its context). Developing this metaphor of the cards on the table, we can see how group purposes fall into four different 'suits'.

♠ Outcomes

Outcomes may relate to individuals in the group, the group as a whole or both. Outcomes concern concrete plans and tasks, and might be described as the group's product, something relatively tangible and measurable. The focus is on the content of group sessions and how these relate to the achievement of individual and group goals. In evidence-based approaches to practice, this is perceived as the 'trump' suit.

♥ Feelings

Groups usually aim to generate feelings of belonging and meaning by fostering mutual respect and support. Individuals bring feelings with them to the group and the group generates its own feelings. Changes in how people feel about themselves are intrinsically linked to changes in their perceptions, attitudes and behaviour. Failure to recognise and work with strong feelings in a group can stymie its progress.

♦ Processes

A group is an opportunity for exchange and mutual aid; groupworkers may hope to develop democratic, participative processes to help people become more empowered, to rehearse new behaviours, to learn new insights. Learning about and using group processes in an open and honest way can help members to become more effective in their personal and social life, as well as helping the group to achieve its aims.

♣ Contexts

All groups take place within a broader context, and it is important that links are made between the inside and the outside of the group. Even in those groups wishing to create a safe haven, the connections to the external environment are important in transferring and generalising the experience in the group to other aspects of group members' lives. There is continual 'trade' between experiences inside and outside the group.

A mnemonic is: ♠ *Specifics;* ♥ *Heart-felts;* ♦ *Dynamics;* ♣ *Contexts*

So, the cards which you present to the group should usually not be confined to one suit. Helen's introduction to the Women of Hope group consisted of feedback from the experience of the individual offers, so her cards were all the more effective because they were ones which had been dealt by the group members themselves:

Women of Hope group
♠ We want to be able to go out alone and be confident
♥ We want to feel whole again
♥ We want to feel good about ourselves
♦ We want to share hidden issues
♣ We want to take control of our own lives and gain acceptance.

Portfolio H, Appendix 1

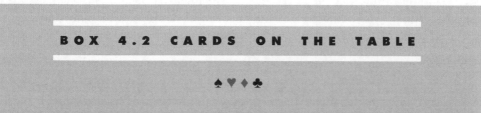

BOX 4.2 CARDS ON THE TABLE

♠ ♥ ♦ ♣

Managing Behaviour for Carers group

In our opening statement, we tried to cover the main aims of the group, which were to look at challenging behaviour from children under the age of 8 years, and to learn new ways for dealing with this behaviour. We went on to say that there is no such thing as a perfect parent and how everyone experiences difficulties at times.

We explained that we felt that, as foster carers, it may be more difficult for them, as the children in their care have come to them with 'learnt behaviour'.

We talked about the child's feelings of confusion and insecurity, and how these feelings may affect the child's behaviour.

We pointed out that it was possible to identify a possibly explosive situation and hopefully defuse it. However, we did recognise that it was not an easy process and situations may get worse before they get better.

We tried to reassure the group that we knew that everyone had their strengths, and we would be building on these, and that the group was there to support each of them along the way.

Portfolio M, 2.3

ACTIVITY 4.3: CARDS ON THE TABLE

Read Mandy's account of the introduction which she and her co-worker, Meg, gave at the beginning of the Managing Behaviour for Carers group (Box 4.2). Consider the four kinds of purpose described earlier (♠ ♥ ♦ ♣) and make a list of 'we wants' for the Managing Behaviour for Carers group in the style of Helen's list for the Women of Hope group (above). Decide which of the four kinds of purpose each 'we want' relates to.

In what ways, and to what extent, do you think the first session (as described in Box 4.3) will have begun to address each of the purposes you have identified?

Mandy wanted to give her group members hope for the possibility of change, but also a realistic understanding that this process would not necessarily be easy:

> We wanted to acknowledge their strengths and offer support to them, but make them aware that the process can be difficult, and may seem to make matters worse at first. This I felt was extremely important if the group members were to persevere with the tactics and strategies.
>
> Portfolio M, 2.3

By attending to the 'red suits', the feelings of hope set against the challenge of the process, Mandy was aiming to increase the chances of a successful outcome.

B O X   4 . 3   F I R S T   S E S S I O N

Managing Behaviour for Carers group

The first session began by Meg and I introducing ourselves. We explained about the Groupwork course, and we asked permission from the group to keep a record of each session, explaining that everything would be anonymised.

The ground rules were then introduced and members were asked if they would like to add any – no-one did.

As an ice-breaker we played the *Name Game*, which worked well, everyone took part and some of the anecdotes were very amusing.

We then went through our 'cards on the table', which included a light-hearted look at the job of the parent/carer *[the cards were reproduced in the portfolio Appendix]*.

Using the flipchart we then did a 'quick think' of the problem behaviour the group members had experienced, both with foster children and their own children. These were then displayed on the wall.

We then took the planned coffee break.

Box 4.3 continued

After coffee we returned to the flipchart and recorded the things that had been tried to address conflict behaviour, and from those, identified what group members felt had worked or not. These again were displayed on the wall *[included in the portfolio Appendix]*.

We then introduced the 'key rules', and as each was explained and discussed it was written up on the flipchart, the group members were given a corresponding handout of the 'key rules' *[reproduced in the portfolio Appendix]*.

Before closing the session, the group members were asked to fill in an anonymous evaluation form *[in the portfolio Appendix]*, which they did.

We then asked if there were any questions, thanked them all for coming and participating and said we would see them next week at the same time.

Portfolio M, 2.3

Commonality and solidarity

> We went on to say that there is no such thing as a perfect parent and how everyone experiences difficulties at times.
>
> Portfolio M, 2.3

One of the oft-mentioned benefits of groupwork is the feeling of all being in the same boat and the sense of normality which this brings. Normalising statements such as Mandy's above can be helpful for group members to begin to position their own experiences in common with others. However, it is equally important that there is no rush to reassure, which can appear to trivialise difficulties and can be experienced by group members as a failure of imagination or comprehension on the groupworkers' part. Comparisons with 'norms' of behaviour in the world outside the group should be made sparingly, while links between the experiences of different members *within* the group should be forged whenever possible. Mandy went on to express her understanding of the particular difficulties which members of the group might face:

> We explained that as foster carers it may more difficult for them, as the children in their care have come to them with 'learnt behaviour'.
>
> Portfolio M, 2.3

As group members begin to put their cards on the table, discussing their own experiences and what they would like from the group, common themes are likely to emerge. The theme of loss through death became apparent in the Women of Hope group. Within the collective experience of the group was the loss of a baby of 7 months in a cot death, the death of a twin child at 3 months, a miscarriage at 2 months, and the loss of a baby through meningitis. There were many other losses of parents and siblings which were also still unresolved.

Helen used a sentence-completion exercise to help group members find common cause and strength. She asked everyone to complete the sentence, *the unhelpful things which people say when you're depressed are …* The Women of Hope group recorded these responses:

- Pull yourself together
- It's all in your head
- You don't need medication
- Why are you like this?
- I know how you feel – I've got the same symptoms
- What have you to worry about?
- What's the matter now?
- Just get your act together.

Portfolio H, Appendix 5

As well as bringing members of the group together in a collective activity, it also helped people to recognise that they were not alone in being the brunt of these opinions, and to share common feelings of frustration and anger. This same sentence-completion technique can be used with most groups, substituting 'depressed' for whatever adjective is most appropriate – ill, in trouble, bereaved, scared, forgetful, etc.

Helen also asked the group early in the first session to consider the positives and negatives of sharing. This kind of activity helps to progress the group in terms of the 'red suits' – feelings (♥) and group process (♦). Again, this is a useful activity whatever the kind of group. This is what the group members recorded:

Positives	Negatives
Relief when we share	What will people think?
It can help to talk	Will anyone care?
Seek out other people's views	Trust could be betrayed
Feeling accepted	Will they understand?
Sharing halves the problem	Will I be judged, rejected, blamed?

Portfolio H, Appendix 6

The outcomes (♠) which group members wish to achieve and the contexts (♣) of their involvement in the group are likely to mark them as different from the group leaders. Of course, groupworkers are concerned about group members achieving successful outcomes, but it is not their (the workers') outcome. In contrast, the 'red suits' are directly shared – group processes are experienced in common, and groupworkers can share their feelings about the group, about the positives and negatives of being in a group for example, alongside other group members. Helen noted that 'The ice-breaker was heavy going initially, but when Harriet [my co-worker] and I participated, it seemed to create a response from some of the group members' (Portfolio H, 3.2).

So, even when the groupworker's situation is very different from group members, they may nevertheless share certain feelings and they will engage in common processes. Orla notes how a feeling of anxiety might arise from different fears, but is nevertheless a shared feeling:

> I shared the feelings of anxiety expressed by most potential group members, but my anxiety centred not around talking in front of the group, but rather

around whether the group would enjoy sessions and take home something positive.

Portfolio O, 6.1

The commonality and solidarity of groups is complex. It should not mask differences, both between workers and members, and between members themselves; individuals coming to the group are likely to come from different starting points. The Sound Start group for young people aged 16 to 17 was designed to help them prepare for independent living. Most, but not all, the group members were in foster homes. Sharleen was in a very settled foster placement and had not really given much thought to moving on. 'Success' for her was beginning to ask questions about what it would be like to leave care, whilst Shelly was just about to move on from her foster placement and was highly receptive to the group's purposes from the start (Portfolio S, 7.2).

Commonality and solidarity can be more difficult to achieve if there is an individual, or a small subgroup of people, whose circumstances are very different to others in the group. For example, a member of the Memory Joggers group had a home carer accompany him to the group initially. How will this person, the home carer, be seen by other group members? Will she be expected to join in group activities and, if not, what will she do during these activities? Individual contacts with people before the group can help alert you to these likely differences and to explore ways in which they may be accommodated.

It may be possible to anticipate some kinds of potential fracture; for example, a mixed-gender group of young people is likely to find itself sitting in two groups, one of boys and another of girls. Group leaders would need to plan how to make use of this likely dynamic, rather than ignore it or try to cajole it away.

JOINING

Once everybody has put their cards on the table, in terms of expressing their hopes and aspirations for the group, the process of joining has already begun (Johnson and Johnson, 1994). A powerful way to build on this experience is to turn the group's attention on itself – how, as a group, should it expect to behave? What guidelines should the group adopt and how is it going to agree these? In short, the group needs to negotiate ground rules.

Ground rules: the group's constitution

There were never any ground rules set and this presented difficulties.

Portfolio F, 2.1

In most cases ground rules should be negotiated during the first meeting of the group, though there may be times when group members need a little longer to get to know each other first. The ground rules are rather like the constitution for the group – a statement of mutual expectations, an agreement about what is acceptable and not acceptable, and possibly what sanctions may be invoked if they are breached. Negotiating the ground rules is a demonstration of care for group processes (♦) and is an important foundation for the group's other purposes.

There are no circumstances which excuse the imposition of pre-written ground rules by the groupworkers. Presenting a group with a list of Do's and Don'ts is not groupwork. Even in groups where members have no choice about attendance – *especially* in these groups – the process of mutual negotiation of the ground rules is a really important rehearsal for participation and developing self-worth. Of course, there may be non-negotiable rules which must be included (for example, no smoking) and groupworkers will play their part in suggesting topics which group members may not have raised, such as confidentiality, but all of this needs to be part of a participative process, as equal as it is possible to be and using the group's vernacular rather than professional language.

It may be necessary to return to the ground rules later in the group's life, when the group members feel more confident to articulate their concerns.

> In establishing ground rules, members were reluctant to put forward their views, perhaps because they were not used to doing this, which had implications for the group being 'theirs'.
>
> Portfolio W, 2.1

Just as 'policy and procedures are crucial as they provide a reference point regarding the roles and responsibilities of professionals' (Horwath and Calder, 1998), so ground rules are a similarly critical reference point for any group.

Confidentiality

It is crucial that 'group members are clear that whatever is discussed should remain within the group and not to be used in idle gossip' (Portfolio F, 3.1). As well as monitoring what goes out of the group, each member should be reminded of their responsibility to consider what comes into the group. The ground rules to which we have referred should emphasise the fact that the privacy of the group does not mean that information has no consequences; disclosure of illegal or dangerous behaviour in the group will have consequences.

Paul and Petra considered wider issues of confidentiality, in terms of trying to build in a degree of anonymity for people coming to the parenting skills group:

> The [group] venue was heavily and continuously used for other activities, so group members would be able to come and go without necessarily identifying themselves as attending a group around 'parenting skills' ... tangible evidence of confidentiality.
>
> Portfolio P, 2.1

It is useful to be reminded that confidentiality is not just about preventing 'idle gossip' but recognising your responsibilities as a groupworker to provide a private space for group participants.

Joining and leaving

The 'classic' group is one where members all join a new group and all say a collective goodbye at the end. However, there are many kinds of group which do not have a first meeting because they are on-going, with people able to join and leave at different times in the group's life. Three of the nine groups illustrating this book fell into this category (the Family Support, Memory Joggers and Offending Awareness groups) and many of the other groups experienced intermittent members who did not necessarily attend every session of the group. As Fran noted,

> We positively encourage new members to the group in order to introduce new ideas and to keep the group as an open membership. I feel this benefits the leaders and existing members alike in that it is less likely to become stale and people are less likely to form cliques.
>
> Portfolio F, 3.1

Orla responded to the practicalities of referrals from the courts to the Offending Awareness group by having new entrants allowed at every fourth session (fortnightly) of the group, when a new topic 'block' began. It worked better than Orla had feared and had some advantages in bringing new spirit into the group, though it did lead to uncertainty about the size of the group, with repercussions on planning group activities. Orla had also supposed that a group of only three would 'get through work more quickly' than a group of ten, but this is not always the case.

Group members' departure at different points is an opportunity to celebrate that person's contribution in a 'graduation' ceremony and also to take stock of the group.

> We reminded the group again that this was Oz's last session and that he was leaving on a positive note by fully completing his court Order. The group was then asked to shout the different feelings which they thought they would have upon finishing their sentence, replacing the usual brainstorm of feelings about the work covered and group participation. We asked Oz to say a few of the feelings he was experiencing and asked him what advice he would offer to the group.
>
> Portfolio O, 6.2

The fact that this session was different, because one of the group's members was leaving, was marked by ending with a game to keep the mood light and, for once, not to go through the usual evaluation sheets. Orla also planned an individual activity chosen by Oz, in this case a tour of a famous football ground.

As I have mentioned, some of those groups that planned for members to join and leave together nevertheless found the need to accommodate late-joiners. The Parents Plus group, often no more than four people including the two co-leaders, was faced by a new member in the sixth of eight sessions, dropped off by her social worker some time after the session had started. The group welcomed the new member and on this occasion the strength of the group proved elastic, capable of stretching to embrace her. This was aided by the fact that the themes which the new member wished to address were similar to those which had already begun to emerge in the group, so the new person's contribution was seen as refreshing this theme, rather than distracting.

If the group has successfully developed an identity as a group, the leaving of a member – planned or unplanned – will usually be a significant event.

> I have noticed that a member permanently leaving the group has a major impact on the remaining members.
>
> Portfolio C, 5.P&O

Teams as groups

Teams are often not seen in groupwork terms and books about teamwork often pay surprisingly scant attention to the groupwork literature (for example, Hutchings *et al.*, 2003). Teams are a type of group whose membership usually joins and leaves at different times, so there is not a 'first' meeting in the way we have been describing in this chapter. For this reason, a team or long-standing working group that wishes to refresh itself must consider carefully how to do this. It is very challenging to work with the team as if it were a new group, but Box 4.4 gives some ideas which can help a team to experience the energy which is engendered by the first meeting of a new group.

If the team is embarking on a new project, or there is an aspect of its work which is changing, this can be a good catalyst for the whole team to consider the benefits of applying groupwork principles to its workings. Few teams negotiate ground rules, for example; without them, many teams suffer and fail to achieve their potential.

BOX 4.4 REFRESHING A TEAM

- Introduce an activity which entails team members saying something new about themselves. For example, the 'Name Game' asks people to introduce themselves by saying how they were given their name, whether it has any particular significance, and what they feel about their name. Disclosing new or different information amongst an established group of people can generate much new energy.
- Consider how to break the pattern of time and place – meeting at a different time and venue or, at the very least, re-arranging the furniture so that team members do not sit as they are accustomed to.
- Change the chairing of the meeting by inviting others to share this task, or invite a consultant to work with the group for an outside perspective.
- Introduce some new and different content to the meeting – perhaps a role-play around a case example from the team's work.

The others

Groups can be in thrall to the power of people who are not actually members of the group, but whose presence is nevertheless felt. A group member might make frequent reference to a partner, to a neighbour or a professional, such as a teacher at their child's school, or their own doctor. Although these characters never enter the stage, they have a proxy membership of the group and can be all the more powerful by their absence. They represent the all-important context for the group (♣) and they should neither be ignored nor treated as a threat. Indeed, they might be 'brought into' the group via role plays and rehearsals. Mandy decided to bring these others into the group by talking about them directly (Activity 4.4). In this case, the others were the children for whom the group members cared. In some groups the others might be invited to make a physical appearance, perhaps as part of the celebrations for the ending.

ACTIVITY 4.4: 'UNSEEN' MEMBERS OF THE GROUP

There are often 'members' of the group who are not present. These are not group members who happen not to be attending this session, but people who never have been members and yet have a presence in the group. For the Managing Behaviour for Carers group these unseen members were the children for whom the group members were caring. Mandy decided to make this explicit with the group:

> We tried to bring the feelings of the children to the group members' attention, as they were 'the unseen members' of the group.
>
> Portfolio M, 2.3

• In what circumstances might it be appropriate to refer to 'unseen' members of the group, and when might it be inappropriate?

Meeting outside the group

Groups should consider what kinds of contact might be appropriate outside its sessions. In addition to meeting potential group members before the group's first session, are there any other circumstances in which a contact outside the group is appropriate? Petra describes how she and co-worker, Paul, contacted individuals by telephone between sessions:

> Each week we [co-leaders] ... telephoned them [group members]. We did this to organise transport, but more importantly to assess how the session had gone for each individual. It was an opportunity to share any difficulties and see how the home task was going.
>
> Portfolio P1, 6.1

If a group member is absent for a session it would normally be appropriate to find out if all is well, and perhaps to let them know what happened in the group to encourage them to attend the following session. Expectations can be discussed when making the group's ground rules – what do we expect the group to do if we miss a session? The group should perhaps also consider in advance what it expects to happen if a group member stops attending.

> Pauline was not mentioned by the others at any point from when she stopped attending ... My sense was that she had felt under pressure to attend from the word go and managed an exit for herself when this possibility occurred; this was never shared with the group.
>
> Portfolio P, 5.1

Of course, group members may well see much of one another between meetings, planned or not. In circumstances where members are likely to have much contact outside the group, you should consider how to bring significant events into the group, perhaps by a check-in at the beginning of the session, inviting comments about contacts since the previous meeting.

KEY POINTS

░ An individual offer of the group to each potential group member has broad benefits.
░ It is important to offer the group in ways which address each individual's particular concerns.
░ Choice and compulsion are complex notions, not polar opposites.
░ Outcomes, feelings, processes and contexts are all significant to the group's life and we should not focus exclusively on outcomes.
░ There are some aspects of the group's life which groupworkers share with group members, and there are other aspects which are unique to the group members.
░ Ground rules provide a solid foundation for the group, and the process of negotiating them helps the various individuals to become a group.

FURTHER READING

Johnson, D.W. and Johnson, F.P. (1994), *Joining Together: Group Theory and Group Skills*, [5th edition], Boston, MA: Allyn and Bacon.
    Chapters 1, 3 and 4 are particularly relevant to the content of this chapter.
Lizzio, A. and Wilson, K. (2001a), 'Facilitating group beginnings: a practice model' in *Groupwork*, 13.1, pp. 6–30, London: Whiting and Birch.
Lizzio, A. and Wilson, K. (2001b), 'Facilitating group beginnings – from basic to working engagement' in *Groupwork*, 13.1, pp. 31–56, London: Whiting and Birch.
    These two articles, in the same issue of *Groupwork*, provide a generic group beginnings model and practice principles to facilitate the forming of groups.
Rooney, R. and Chovanec, M. (2004), 'Involuntary groups' in C.D. Garvin, L.M. Gutiérrez and M.J. Galinsky (eds), *Handbook of Social Work with Groups*, pp. 212–26, New York: Guilford Press.
    This chapter focuses specifically on the issue of choice and working with people who are not voluntary members of the group.
Shulman, L. (1999) *The Skills of Helping Individuals, Families, Groups and Communities* [4th edition], Itasca, IL: Peacock.
    This remains a classic text and is particularly helpful in terms of preparation and concepts such as 'tuning in' to groups.

FOOTNOTE

1 In fact, it comes from the Women of Hope group (Box 1.H).

CHAPTER 5

DO

OBJECTIVES

By the end of this chapter you should be able to:

- Work together with group members to design group sessions
- Improvise and allow appropriate 'unplanned' time for the group
- Use a wide range of group methods and techniques with groups
- Help groups to develop a sense of group identity
- Enable groups to feel creative and develop their sense of playfulness.

In this chapter we will consider what groups do and what they are capable of doing. For the groupworker in particular, but for all group members, there is an element of performance in groups, and I have used a theatrical metaphor to present the material in the first section of the chapter.

STAGING THE GROUP

The cast, the set, the props

In previous chapters we have considered how best to bring group members together, the significance of the setting for the group and the need to prepare the necessary props to resource and equip the group (see Box 3.4). Even when the cast is decided, gathering it together is sometimes a prelude to the drama, as Jenny regularly experienced with the Memory Joggers group:

> Service users would forget what days we would be coming to collect them; it took time locking up their homes; they would forget bags, keys, even teeth and we would have to go back for them; some had poor mobility and would struggle getting in and out of cars; and carers would want to spend time talking as we were leaving with the service user.
>
> Portfolio J, 2.1

Scripts

There are two ways in which the concept of script is useful in groupwork. The first is the notion of 'life scripts' developed by Eric Berne through transactional analysis and the 'Games People Play' (Berne, 1967). The insights which people can gain from an understanding of the ways in which their lives are scripted can help them break from the script and rehearse new roles. Learning about scripts with others in a group makes this journey less lonely.

There is another way in which this notion of script is enlightening: the notion of the group's script. To what extent are you writing the script for the group, indeed, using someone else's material (with 'off-the-shelf' groups) and to what extent is the group increasingly writing its own? We need to know more about how, when and whether scripted groups might work well.

Improvising

Most groups are likely to have some degree of scripting, in the sense that there is form and structure to the group session. In groups which have been created by professionals there will be an expectation that they exercise their leadership by planning what the group will do (see Box 3.4). In their attention to group process, leaders should always be looking for opportunities to share the scripting with group members, indeed, to encourage the membership's confidence and ability to take on this responsibility, depending on what is realistic to expect.

Even the most closely scripted group should allow group members time to respond and make use of the material, though the degree to which the group has manoeuvre to depart from plan and to improvise varies. There are two different triggers for improvisation. The first is responding to an immediate crisis or unplanned event in the group, sometimes around a 'prop' failure, but more likely as a result of the unexpected behaviour of one particular member of the group. Jenny's description of Jean's agitation (Box 5.1) is such an example – and note how the workers involve the whole group in this. The second is not a sudden event, but perhaps a change in the group's mood or responses which suggests the need to depart from plan.

> Most of the session happened as planned except during the first half when the group members were getting bored and switching off. We had planned for this eventuality and we introduced a tower-building competition with newspaper and sellotape to energise them.
>
> Portfolio S, 4.1

In this same group, a game of Chinese whispers designed to begin a session around the theme of communication was not working because the young people found it impossible to whisper! They extemporised and decided that the 'whisper' had to be passed on from outside the room, which worked both for the purpose of demonstrating the effect of miscommunication and maintaining interest through the physical activity. It also demonstrated the group's problem-solving ability.

Heavily scripted group sessions can focus so much on the content of the session that the group's *response* to this content is neglected. Wendy recognised this when she reflected on the summing up at the end of the group, and the difference between a reiteration of the information provided and a summary of group members' experiences and learning:

> There was the usual summing up at the end. However, this session was different in that as co-workers, we did not hold the power in terms of [pre-] knowledge of the content of the session. Thus the summing up at the end involved seeing everyone's personal experiences as valid forms of information, whereas in more planned sessions, a lot of the summing up involved re-emphasizing factual information ... this seemed to be one of the sessions which stuck in group members' minds most.
>
> Portfolio W, 6.2

BOX 5.1   IMPROVISING

Memory Joggers group – Jean arrives agitated

Jean arrived at the group agitated and upset. Whenever she is agitated she becomes confused and disorientated. She struggled to get her fleece off, so Julie helped her and sat her comfortably in a chair. I brought Jean a drink of tea and asked her how she was feeling. She immediately said, 'It's him again!' By this time most of the other members were settled down and several asked her if she was alright'. Jean explained that she had been arguing with her husband and that 'he was taking his bad mood out on me'. Apparently he has rushed her that morning and complained about how long it took her to get ready. I asked Jean if his back was playing him up again. When he is in pain he is less tolerant and understanding of Jean's situation.

She confirmed that he was in the middle of decorating the house and refused to rest up until it was all finished. I said it was very frustrating when decorating because even when doing only one room, the whole house tends to be disrupted. This opened up a discussion with other group members. Julie said that this had probably triggered off his back pain and that he was probably doing too much. Jean agreed and said she'd told him, but 'he won't listen'. Jane, one of the group members, said 'you're better off here then, out of his way'. By this time Jean, who had received support and reassurance from the group, was able to laugh it off and joked about it being 'his problem, not mine – oh, leave him to it'.

Portfolio J, 4.3

Beware improvisations which merely fill gaps. Jenny recognised that this occurred in the Memory Joggers group when there had not been sufficient planning for a session and they fell back on bingo. Although this is an activity which group members enjoyed, it offered no added value.

ACTIVITY 5.1: WHAT HAPPENS NEXT?

Westville Women's group
We had originally planned for two members of the Community Police to take the session, having found out through a local resource centre that they offered short workshops on 'women and safety'. However, they had to pull out that morning due to an emergency and had left us the video.

Portfolio W, 6.2

You have 30 minutes before the group is due to start. What would you do next in these circumstances?

Timing and pace

As with theatre, groupwork depends on good timing. When to ask the group to work on its ground rules, at what point to focus on a difficult or taboo subject, and when to suggest a new kind of activity are all matters of judgement which groupworkers make on the basis of their experience with previous groups and their antennae with the current one. You cannot always be successful.

> The women were fairly reluctant to put forward their contributions [at this early stage of the first group session] – perhaps they had never negotiated a group contract before. With hindsight, I think we should have referred back to the contract at the end of the session, when the women were more relaxed.
>
> Portfolio W, 3.3

You should try to vary the pace of a group, because this will tend to make it more stimulating, like varying the pitch and tone of one's voice. Individuals tend to have difference preferences around pace, so variation helps to keep most people on board most of the time.

Prompts

Many of the activities which are used in groups are designed as prompts to move the group on. Open discussion can be dominated by the more articulate or verbal members of the group, and it can wander. Prompts help to bring focus to a discussion, and they can be introduced in ways which encourage wider participation. For example, if each group member has their own prompt on a card there can be an expectation that each will share their own prompt. Depending on how imaginative the group is, you may sometimes consider providing example responses to prompts. Prompts can be used to alter the pace of the group, to quicken or to slow it.

There may be other reasons for prompts in the group. For example, the visual prompt of writing on a whiteboard was especially appreciated by the Memory Joggers group. This group also used olfactory prompts – smells – to help people's memories, and 'because group members have memory problems we find ourselves doing a shortened version of the Opening Statement of Purpose every week to remind them what the group is all about' (Portfolio J, 3.3).

ACTIVITY 5.2: DESIGNING PROMPTS

Crimestop group

Which is worse? The innocent being punished or the guilty going free?

Choose three of the groups below and design a similar, brief prompt designed to spark discussion and controversy around a topic appropriate to each of the groups you have chosen. Why do you think your prompt would be likely to stimulate discussion?

Family Support group   *Offending Awareness group*
Women of Hope group   *Parents Plus group*
Memory Joggers group   *Sound Start group*
Managing Behaviour group   *Westfield Women's group.*

Refer to Boxes 1.C to 1.W (pages 9–20) if you need to refresh your memory of these groups.

Plots and sub-text

The main plot for any group is usually obvious and will have been the focus of the offer of groupwork to potential members early on – 'Offending Awareness', 'Family Support', for example. Initially, this main plot is likely to be the principal guide for the group's activities. For example, in the Sound Start group, Samantha used the theme of moving from care to independent living to construct an activity for the whole group to take part in:

> [In Storyboard] each member had a large piece of paper divided into ten squares. They had to draw themselves at different times throughout a typical day; sleeping, eating, going to college, being with friends, etc. They then had to attach pre-prepared stickers to identify which basic needs they had met during the day; e.g. food, shelter, warmth, friendship.
>
> Portfolio S, 4.2

This kind of activity can help make connections between group members, in terms of common themes in their lives, and it can also open up potential areas of difference, which gives the group the opportunity to rehearse working with these differences.

Unexpected commonalities can emerge, such as the shared interest in music amongst members of the Sound Start group, which also gave them something separate from the group leaders. Other themes will often develop out of the main plot; like a story unfolding, sub-texts begin to surface, sometimes with the direct encouragement of the groupworkers but often spontaneously.

Workers in the Groupwork Project (Box 1.1) were trained to identify and note themes as they began to emerge, and Paul made this record of the work of the Parents Plus group:

> After session 4, I recorded two particular themes which were emerging. The first was domestic violence. The second was the significance of other adults; by this I meant that former partners were able to exert significant influence from a distance ... the unpredictability of men.
>
> Portfolio P, 5.3

A sub-plot in the Offending Awareness group was the fact that all the members had themselves been victims of crime and 'many of the young people appeared surprised by this common theme' (Portfolio O, 5.3). Orla also noted a sense of loss as another sub-text, though it was not explicitly named: loss of positive family relationships, loss of a stable home, loss of freedom to attend education or employment due to criminal record, etc.

> For many members, some form of loss may have been the trigger for some of their offending, whilst for others it may be a consequence of their involvement with the Criminal Justice system.
>
> Portfolio O, 5.3

The significance of these themes is their power to bring individuals in the group together, to move from a set of individuals to a *group*, and to help the group gain a better insight of the main plot. Groupworkers need to be sensitive to the emergence of sub-text in the group, which means helping the group to uncover it, whilst not aggressively digging for it.

The interval

Most groups plan a break. Although the group usually sees this as 'time out', in fact it is very much a part of the group process. It might be used to digest what has just been experienced in the group, or to test out some unexpressed thoughts and feelings with a trusted person. Even when the talk is of entirely different matters – 'talents, interests and hobbies' (Sharry, 1999: 79) – this, too, gives group members a rounder picture of one another. For the groupworker the break can be a good time to check out an individual member about whom there is concern, or just to leave the rest of the group out of their gaze, as Petra reflected with hindsight:

> What I feel hinders the process is that Paul [my co-worker] and I sat with the group in the break. I think this stops the group members talking to each

other and prevents them from making personal links away from the group. Part of our aim was to encourage contact outside the group.

Portfolio P1, 6.1

Providing refreshments is a tangible expression of the care which the groupworkers feel for the group. Nurturing the group in this way can feel especially significant if the workers have had to be particularly challenging or have pressed the group to work with stressful matters.

> [It] gave members a sense of being valued; the drinks were brought in for their use, and served by the group leaders which had a slight feel of pampering.
>
> Portfolio P, 6.1

It would seem disrespectful of a group's needs not to plan a break, yet one of the greatest mistakes in meetings is to plough on regardless. Indeed, if meetings could be treated as group sessions, we would see better practices. A good rule of thumb is to have a ten-minute break after every hour of meeting. The physical movement is beneficial in itself, the break enables people to see to personal needs (smoke, loo, coffee), to back away from entrenched positions, to sound others out informally and to reposition (physically as well as metaphorically).

Leaving the stage

The break is an opportunity for the whole group to leave the stage, and it is worthwhile considering the circumstances when it might be appropriate for just one or two members to exit before the end – sometimes called 'time out'. This might mean physically leaving the group room, or just exercising a right to opt out of an activity. This is something which the group should discuss as part of its ground rules; however, it is a complex topic, so it may be something to review once the group is established.

Individuals who consistently withhold are often seen as hindering the group's work or unfairly not contributing; on the other hand, some people may be emotionally or intellectually less able to contribute. It may be a question of 'from each according to their abilities and to each according to their needs', which could be a good focus for the group's discussion. In a group where attendance is obligatory, allowing more choice and opt out within the group may be one way of compensating for the larger lack of choice. Moreover, it may be an opportunity to find that person an additional or new role:

> Only one person chose not to be filmed because of nerves but as it had been agreed by the group that this was acceptable if someone felt uncomfortable, it caused few problems. The young person who chose not to be filmed was asked to take on the job of holding up prompt cards for the 'actors' to read from.
>
> Portfolio O, 4.1

Even so, when reflecting on this individual's part, Orla felt he had 'not felt the same sense of achievement as the others' (Portfolio O, 4.1).

Rehearsal – and applause

There are two kinds of rehearsal which the group might use. The first involves the whole group and takes place during the group session, in the way described by Orla in the previous section. The strength and support of the group is used to try out new ways of thinking, feeling and behaving. The second kind involves individuals rehearsing their learning from experiences within the group in their 'real' worlds. Reporting these between-sessions experiences often provides the material for the beginning of the subsequent group meeting; sharing triumphs or receiving consolation, helps support group members either to move on to the next stage, or to re-rehearse.

Even when it is obvious how an improvement could be made, it is sometimes only when this has been rehearsed with the group that a person feels ready or able to put it into practice. Learning techniques such as 'the pause button', then putting them quickly into practice and seeing immediate returns can be the most positive experience a group member has had for some time.

> Pat was pleased with herself: 'I can't believe how I handled Peter [her son] yesterday'. In her excitement, the story tumbled out. She was called back from a social gathering to be confronted on her doorstep by a Police Officer. Peter had been involved in some troublesome activity, he wasn't being charged but was being warned. After the officer left, Pat listened to Peter with growing impatience and anger. When he finished, she said, 'I'm really angry with you, too angry to think what I should do so I'm going to think about this and when I'm ready we are going to sort this out.' Pat was delighted both with Peter's response, as this had clearly made an impact, as well as her sister's response: 'I can't believe how well you've dealt with that.' Pat views her sister's approach to parenting as 'top drawer', so this was praise indeed.
>
> Portfolio P, 5.2

On tour

Groups need to consider whether to leave the relative safety and familiarity of their usual venue and venture out. Whatever the reasons for the group's change of venue and activities, an outside visit invariably shows the group and its individual members (and the group leaders) in a different light. Wendy relates a situation in which the whole group could help one of its members rehearse a new skill, supporting her physically and emotionally, in a way that would be impossible in the group's usual venue.

> In one session the group visited the Westville Dome to take part in a Women's Day, which included swimming, sauna and jacuzzi. Wanda was very nervous. She had not been in water for over 20 years and was very fearful. However, she still wanted to go ahead with the visit to try it out. Group members … offered words of encouragement, relating their own fears in order to make

her not feel alone, and physically assisting Wanda by holding her up [in the water]. Wanda gained a lot of confidence from this experience and took part in all the activities. It increased her self-esteem and she expressed a wish to take adult swimming lessons.

Portfolio W, 5.2

A trip is often organised as the finale to a group, but it may be better to plan this as the penultimate session, so that the final meeting can take place in the familiar territory of the group room.

Curtain – transitional activities

We had to clear the room prior to a relatively quick departure, which effectively 'tidied the room away' for us – it was a definite conclusion to a session for ourselves as group leaders.

Portfolio P, 6.1

One of the groupworker's tasks is time-keeping, and this is especially significant as the group session nears its end. Establishing a pattern for endings helps the group as a whole to learn to pace itself; the relaxation exercises used in the Women of Hope group became the signal that the group was nearing its end (Box 3.4). This kind of transitional activity helps to prepare group members to leave, so that they are not caught by the curtain dropping without warning. Transitional activities also help the group to avoid the curtain becoming 'stuck', as Paul describes in Box 5.2 below. We can all sympathise with this predicament, especially common in those team meetings where people feel at liberty to come and go early and late, and there is no transition. When people finally leave, there is a sense of frustration. A regular transitional activity prevents this.

Those which are open-ended, like the Family Support and Memory Joggers groups, should plan their own curtain calls at regular intervals, perhaps every three or so months, so that the group or team can take stock and re-group accordingly. These sessions should be marked out as different from others, perhaps by revisiting the ground rules, completing written evaluations and making plans for the next period in the group's life.

An audience?

The theatre metaphor breaks down when we consider that plays are presented for the entertainment of others, whilst the group's stage is private and curtained off. However, some social action groups will be oriented towards a wider audience, and there is good cause for other kinds of group to consider whether there is, in fact, an 'audience' and how it might be involved in the group's work. In Chapter 4 we considered the context for the group (♣) and the others who may not be members of the group but have an influence. If this is an especially significant factor, the group should consider whether and how to bring this potential audience into the group itself.

BOX 5.2 WHEN THE CURTAIN GETS STUCK

Parents Plus – role play

At length, we introduced the topic of the day, 'active listening'. We role played; my co-leader was the stroppy adolescent, I was the concerned parent re-framing the content of my daughter's verbal attack by being attentive to the feelings underlying this. Penny and Pat agreed to try this: Pat was initially the loud teenager, Penny the concerned parent, and Penny immediately grasped the idea and was an excellent active listener.

   Roles reversed, Penny became the not-too-demanding youngster, Pat the concerned listener. It was clear from the start that Pat struggled with the concept, offering desperate solutions at each turn while Penny, for her part, supportively became increasingly accommodating.

   Time was moving on, already ten minutes from the end of the session and no hot drinks. My co-leader went to reception to be told they had forgotten. We cobbled together an ending using the drinks machine and available biscuits as the taxis arrived to return people home.

Portfolio P, 4.1

ACTIVITY 5.3: AUDIENCE PARTICIPATION

It is rare for a group to open its doors to others who have not been members, yet the impact of the group on others can be substantial. Also, direct contact with the group by people in a position to support further groups can increase awareness and help to sustain and develop groupwork as a service.

   For each of the nine groups which illustrate this book, another group of people is suggested below for possible attendance at a special session of the group. Choose three of the groups and consider the possible purposes of them meeting with the group, and the advantages and disadvantages of this. If the advantages outweigh the disadvantages, and assuming that the group itself is agreeable, plan a session of the group to include this 'invited audience'.

Crimestop group	*Offending Awareness group*
Magistrates	Victims of crime
Family Support group	*Parents Plus group*
Local council officials	The group members' children
Women of Hope group	*Sound Start group*
Family or friends	Current carers (foster parents; residential workers)

Memory Joggers group
Partners and carers

Westfield Women's group
Other professionals from the team

Managing Behaviour group
Agency managers

Refer to Boxes 1.C to 1.W (pages 9–20) to refresh your memory of these groups.

METHODS AND TECHNIQUES

The terms methods and techniques tend to be used interchangeably. However, we might distinguish 'methods' as specific interventions, such as those in Box 5.3 suggested to help to develop group identity. Each method would entail the use of a number of techniques, such as accurate listening, pointing to inconsistencies, negotiating and the like (Bertcher, 1994). I have detailed elsewhere, with Catherine Sawdon, a wide range of 'action techniques' (Doel and Sawdon, 1999a, ch. 7). In the space available here I will focus on methods and techniques which can be used to promote what is a central process in groupwork – helping a set of individuals to become a group.

Talking and listening

Groups talk. Indeed, open or semi-structured discussion is probably the most common of group activities. This detailed account of an episode in the Women of Hope group testifies to the importance of talk.

> Hazel shared with the group her terrible fear of dying ... her mother died of a stroke when Hazel was 17 and Hazel fears the same will happen to her ... I asked the group if death was an issue for them ... Harmony had similar fears, whilst Hannah said death had always been an issue for her and she has only recently let her mother go despite the fact that she had been dead for a number of years. She said she neglected her family because she could only focus on her dead mother ... I asked Hazel if she had used any methods to deal with her fears. She said she could not, it was too difficult ...
>
> Portfolio H, 4.2

In fact, talking is only one side of the equation. Whilst an individual talks, the group listens. When another individual takes on the talk, the group continues its listening: except that the individuals may need to learn to talk and the group may need to learn to listen. Your groupwork should focus on how best to facilitate this.

Group identity

> During early sessions, Oscar would say 'I think that …' despite feeding back joint ideas from working in a pair. After attending several sessions, Oscar began to feed back in the plural, '*We* think that …'.
>
> Portfolio O, 5.3

A key notion in the transformation from a set of individuals to a group is *identity*. Achieving a sense of group identity is unlikely to be named as an explicit aim, but without this transformation the named outcomes are less likely to be achieved. Paul, co-leader of the Parents Plus group, acknowledged the difficulty of moving from a set of individuals to a group when he viewed the video-tape of one of the sessions.

> The extract has a sense of individual counselling rather than being a group. All attention was focused in one person's direction. What would have been better would be to have acknowledged others in the room without them needing to speak up to be 'seen'.
>
> Portfolio P, 9.1

In contrast, Fran describes how the members of the Family Support group pitched in to re-decorate the group's meeting place, a kind of feathering of the group's nest which helped to develop a sense of the group working together (Portfolio F, 4.2). People had different roles and contributed at different levels, but this mutual activity helped the group to identity itself *as a group*.

There is some evidence from the Groupwork Project (Box 1.1) that groupworkers find it easier to work with individuals in the group than to help the group develop its identity as a group. Interactions and techniques which focused on the group as a group are less in evidence than those which were aimed at individuals in sequence. The suggested activities in Box 5.3 can accelerate the process of group identity. In particular, a group can very quickly develop a sense of its identity by story-telling, which creates 'a moral gymnasium in which limbering up can take place' (Fairbairn, 2002: 23).

BOX 5.3 GROUP IDENTITY

Eight ways to develop group identity

Choose a name
Often the name of the group has been a 'given', but choosing a name for the group *as a group* is an excellent way for the group to consider what it stands for.

Sentence completion
Have the group focus on itself as a group by answering sentences which begin: 'In this group I feel …'; 'This group helps us to …'; 'If this group were a colour it would be … '; 'I would like other people to see this group as …'

Box 5.3 continued

Scarce resource game
The group is in competition with three other groups for a much desired prize (tailor this to the particular group). The group must build a case as to why it deserves the prize more than any other group. You can leave these other groups as unknowns, or supply details for them.

Group tangle
The group holds hands in a circle. Then, by stepping over and ducking under the arms of people opposite, and not letting go of any hands, the group knots itself until it cannot move any more. Then the group must untangle itself without letting go of any hands.

Re-decorating
The group's meeting room is up for redecoration and the group must choose a colour scheme and new furnishings. It's great if the group can actually do this, but even a hypothetical re-decoration plan can be very effective to build group identity.

Coat of arms
The group must decide on its coat of arms. Once the group has discussed and agreed what this should look like, it sets to with coloured paper, paints and the like to make one. The group then reflects on why and how this coat of arms was chosen.

Docudrama
The group is being featured in a Channel 4 docudrama, 'What makes a group?' The groupworkers interview the group for an in-depth, inside look at what makes the group work.

The group symbolised by an animal
'If this group were an animal, what kind of an animal would it be?' Everyone has to make a case for their own 'animal', and then the group negotiates which of these to choose as its emblem.

ACTIVITY 5.4: DEVELOPING GROUP IDENTITY

Consider each of the eight suggestions for building group identity (Box 5.3). Do some of these methods seem more appropriate early in the group's life and others later – when there is already some group identity established?

List the methods in order, starting with those you would be most likely to use early in the group's life and finishing with those you would use later.

Although talking and listening are probably the most significant techniques in the process of transformation from individuals to a group, there are many other effective ways of enhancing and accelerating this process.

Writing and reading

The discussion about fears in the Women of Hope group came to an impasse with further discussion proving too difficult, certainly for group member Hazel. At this point, groupworker Helen suggests a different medium, writing, to unstick the group.

> I asked Hazel if she had used any methods to deal with her fears. She said she could not, it was too difficult … I suggested the possibility of writing down a plan of action as if she was speaking to the other members of her family who could make arrangements for her in the event of her death … Hazel and the group felt this was a good idea and we began to draw up a plan.
>
> Portfolio H, 4.2

With the provisos around levels of literacy, knowledge of English and visual ability, written techniques are very adaptable in groups. The group's thoughts and feelings can be collected together spontaneously on a collective sheet of flipchart paper and re-visited later; pre-written sheets can be introduced into the group; letters can be created, either by the group as a whole or by each member, perhaps writing a letter to themselves which will be opened later in the group's life. A single word or phrase on a card can trigger discussion; questionnaires and evaluation sheets can help the group take its own pulse; information sheets can be taken away for people to read in their own time.

Introducing a written format into the group usually helps slow the pace a little; people can reflect on how the flipchart is building up, they can deliberate over their letter, cross out and re-do responses on the evaluation sheet as they re-think them. Written materials can be read later, providing a ready record of the group's life, and a useful reminder, for example of the ground rules.

Orla noted how the introduction of 'dry' written statistics helped to provide initial distance to a topic which she knew the group members would find difficult. Distancing techniques help people begin to circle around a subject before landing on it, and material in written format can provide additional distance.

> As group leaders we were apprehensive about exploring intimate issues [such as sexual health] with the group members and we felt that the use of statistics achieved the purpose of allowing group members, and us, to become more comfortable with the topic before deeper discussion.
>
> Portfolio O, 4.2

Fran describes how random written cards helped the group articulate feelings which it might not otherwise have chosen to do:

> We have 'feelings cards' and a member can pick out a card to discuss with us what they feel about the group, e.g. a card may read 'SAFE', and a member might then say, 'I feel safe within this group because …'
>
> Portfolio F, 7.2

There are, of course, a host of other methods not specifically related to talking, listening, reading or writing – such as art work (Argyle and Bolton, 2004; St Thomas and Johnson, 2002) – which we do not have space to explore. However, I shall move on to consider how all methods and techniques build patterns for groups, and the significance of both making and breaking these patterns.

Making and breaking patterns

Group identity is related to a sense of consistency. Each time the group meets it adds to its own history, developing in-jokes which make reference to itself based on its experience of past sessions. As individuals in the group begin to know one another better they settle into a pattern of relationships and expectations of what the group will and can do.

Much of this patterning comes from the format of the group. The regularity of its time and place of meeting and the pace and style of what it does, all contribute to growing familiarity. Warm-ups, check-ins, breaks, exercises, ending rituals are used as what Paul described as 'punctuation', and group members come to expect this in each session. From one session to the next, people start to sit in the same chair, occupying 'their' space. Even a short-lived group is likely to develop traditions:

> While the quality of the video clips was not the highest order, the use of these had the effect of punctuating sessions that was helpful … The pre-written flipcharts have been used at all groups and, therefore, have an element of tradition about them.
>
> Portfolio P, 4.2

Group identity can transcend changing membership, as Orla discovered with the Offending Awareness group, in which there were new entrants every fourth session. Old hands found themselves inducting the new recruits into the existing patterns (see Box 5.4).

> The more experienced group members would explain the session layout and expectations to new members, signifying a change from feelings of uncertainty to those of familiarity and belonging.
>
> Portfolio O, 3.2

Groups enjoy different degrees of familiarity. A group such as Memory Joggers relied heavily on establishing patterns to help group members to exercise their short-term memory and sustain it. As members grew more comfortable with one another from session to session, they were less embarrassed by their difficulties and more willing to take risks.

Breaking patterns

Towards the end of one of the more emotive sessions of the Offending Awareness group, Orla felt it was important to allow group members time to debrief. However, she discovered how difficult in can be to break a pattern once it has become fixed.

BOX 5.4 FAMILIARITY

Offending Awareness group

It was hoped that familiarity [with the pattern of each session] would help to alleviate concerns of members.

Each session therefore was planned to open with:

- a warm welcome to the group and introductions to new and existing members
- a fun warm-up (e.g. young people and leaders asked to write down one true and one false statement about themselves which they are OK to share, then go round the group deciding which was true and which was false)
- code of conduct/group rules agreed/reviewed
- introduction as to why it was important to explore the topic of the session
- a brief outline of session content and activities planned
- regular breaks, to accommodate relatively low attention span of some members
- the main session content and activities
- final summary of work completed and discussion of how the session went
- evaluation by the group members of the session
- bus fare and travel arrangements dealt with.

Portfolio O, 3.2

This unfamiliar element of the session ending was the least successful [of our endings]. The group recognized from previous sessions that evaluation signalled the end of discussion and the opportunity to obtain travel fares. My co-worker and I then had to work very hard to regain the attention of the group to address the highly important area [of debriefing] before everyone dispersed.

Portfolio O, 6.1

It is one of the many paradoxes in groupwork that, whilst establishing patterns is such a significant method of developing group identity, it is just as important to know when and how to break a pattern to prevent it from inhibiting group progress. Rather like physical exercise, where initial gains can plateau as the body gets used to the new regime, so the pattern that was helpful when the group was starting out can become outmoded for its current purposes. These tendencies are especially prevalent in team meetings and often remain unchecked, perhaps because team meetings are so seldom conceptualised as group sessions.

Patterns may be broken spontaneously, as events inside or outside the group provoke change, or the groupworkers might plan something different. This usually entails taking a calculated risk, as Wendy found when introducing activities which the women in the Westville Women's group had probably not experienced since their childhoods. These included 'Fruit Salad', a variant on musical chairs which the women 'all joined in enthusiastically' (Portfolio W, 3.2).

New kinds of activity are usually introduced into the group to shift to a different level. The group might reconstruct its identity by re-thinking its name: 'The group's always been called the X group, but what do we think of this? Is this the right name for our group, or can we think of one that would be even more fitting?'

Mandy and her co-worker, Meg, decided to introduce role play into the Managing Behaviour for Carers group, though it was clear that the group members were apprehensive and found this demanding. However, in the subsequent, anonymous evaluations they indicated that they were all pleased to have taken part and learned much from it. Perhaps most instructive of all, it encouraged one of the group members to take a giant stride in the 'quick-think' which followed the role plays:

> I became aware that Meera was not participating and in fact looked ill at ease. When I asked her if she had anything to say, she replied, 'I'll be glad when he goes' [her foster child], and then added, 'that sounds awful, doesn't it?' Everyone supported Meera in her feelings and the comment was added to the flipchart with all the others.
>
> Portfolio M, 3.2

The new activity (role play) had put appropriate pressure on the group, provoking a sense of achievement and closeness which helped Meera to express feelings which were different from all the other group members, as she saw it, and generally ones which would be seen as unacceptable outside the group. It gave the group as a whole the opportunity to show its collective support for her.

There are other patterns which group members are often hoping to break – the patterns of feelings and behaviours that are experienced outside the group and which are often the motivation for being in the group. The challenge for the groupworker is how to ensure that it is the new behaviours and roles within the group that are reinforced outside the group, and not the behaviours which have been established outside the group that continue to be re-played within it.

Creativity and playfulness

Above all else, the experience of groupwork should be creative. The development of an identity as a group should be qualitatively different from the experience of solo working. In addition to all the benefits of working together in groups it is this opportunity for creativity which is so much more pronounced in a group. It is often released through play. Play, and the resulting playfulness, makes the group a different experience.

I use 'play' in its broadest sense. It is about fun and spontaneity, performing and even pretending, and learning about fair play, rules and participation. Play can be frivolous, but it can also allow a group to approach and deal with difficult and painful topics. An example of this is the Links activity (Boxes 3.4 and 5.5), which permits the topics in question to be light or heavy, remote or personal. Groupwork methods are often designed to liberate the group's sense of playfulness and, like the best plays, the mood can swing swiftly from comedy to tragedy and back.

Playfulness is assisted by movement. The Links activity is an example of this. Group members are in continual motion, up and down the imaginary line, crossing and re-crossing one another's paths, forming and re-forming different subgroups along the length of the line. Individual group members develop different perspectives of each other, both literally and metaphorically. Physical movement is significant, but this does not mean that people with mobility problems are excluded from developing playfulness. For example, in the Links method, wheelchair users can position their chairs along the line; people with considerable mobility limitations can participate by pointing at a line drawn on flipchart paper to represent the imaginary line across the room. Groupworkers and members must all work hard to ensure that methods and techniques are inclusive.

The groupworker's skill is to help the group reflect on the experiences generated by a method or technique and to relate these to experiences both within the group and outside it, in people's lives beyond the group. In essence, this is what makes what could be a meaningless activity into a groupwork *method*. Moreover, we will see in the next chapter that no method is neutral or without its context (see Activity 6.5, Follow my leader).

BOX 5.5 GETTING PHYSICAL

Westville Women's group – 'Links'

We have used the Links game* on a number of occasions. In the first session we used it twice. First we had lighthearted topics, such as 'hairy chests' and 'bikinis'. The game helped break the ice and got the women moving around. It also helped promote discussion of reasons for people's dislikes, and emphasized similarities and differences.

In the same session we used the Links game to decide on the two group activities which the group would do in later sessions. We had already brainstormed people's ideas, written these on cards, and used these for the Link game. I think that, without the aid of the game, the women would have been reluctant to express their preference, especially at such an early stage of the group's life. However, by using the Links game, which is active, the women were able to be vocal about their preferences and also provoked discussion. The method proved very effective.

We also used the Links game as part of the stress management session, where potentially stressful situations were written on the cards and the group members had to demonstrate their likes and dislikes.

Portfolio W, 4.2

* In the **Links** game (sometimes called Continuum), people are asked to position themselves along an imaginary line running diagonally across the room. One end of the line represents strongly held likes, the other end strongly held dislikes, with gradations in between (the middle signifying 'take it or leave it'). When a topic is read out, everyone positions themselves along the line according to how much they love or loathe it. This is followed by discussion of the topic itself and also reflection on the different 'links' that are forged and broken as people re-position themselves. Group members find out more about one another and new groupings of opinion are usual from topic to topic. The groupworkers can write the topics beforehand, or group members can compose them. (Writing the topics on cards, shuffling and dealing out to everyone in the group maintains anonymity of each topic's author.)

BOX 5.6 ICE-BREAKERS, WARM-UPS, COOL-DOWNS

Introductions and name-learning

Name games
In a circle, throw a soft ball to each other, calling your own name and the person you throw to (Mary to Yusef ... Yusef to Gail, etc.)
Each person talks about their own name, what it means to them.
Introduce your neighbour – chance for group leaders to model the kind of information which should be shared by breaking into pairs.
Breakfast game – 'I'm Diane and for breakfast I had ...'; 'I'm Carol and for breakfast I had ... and that is Diane and she had ...' and so on.

Starting conversation

Newspapers – recent clippings are used to generate discussion.
Personal news – something that has happened to you since the last session.

Active- energising warm-ups

Joan of Arc – a famous person's name is stuck on your back – the rest of group has to mime who it is until you guess.
Fruit Salad – each person is a member of a set of fruit (so there are 4–5 oranges, 4–5 apples, etc.) – there's one chair too few and the person in the middle calls a fruit and all those fruits have to change seats. Person left in the middle calls name of fruit, etc. Calling 'Fruit salad' means everyone must move.
Jungle Book – each person is a jungle animal with their own action; one person is the skunk and tries to catch you out by calling your name. If you don't do your action before the skunk, you become the skunk.
Keeper of the keys – blindfolded person in centre has to listen out for person attempting to steal the keys and point successfully at where the 'thief' is.
Get into order – participants string themselves along a line according to, say, birthdays; for example by miming horoscopes.
Elimination games:
Shipwreck / balloon debate, etc. – group members take on a role (lawyer, painter–decorator, hairdresser, teacher, etc.) and have to argue their case as to why they are needed to survive.
Killer – the killer winks at his/her victims, who then becomes the killer.

We're all in this together; physical contact

Machine – small subgroups go off to choose a piece of moving domestic machinery, rehearse how to mime it, then perform it for the rest of the group who must guess what it is.

Box 5.6 continued

Sharks – group members have to leap on to an improvised mat in the middle of the room when 'shark!' is called. The mat is made progressively smaller. The whole group lose sif any one member is eaten by the shark.
Trust games – in pairs, one partner is blindfolded and the other partner leads him/ her around.
Lemons – each member brings their own lemon, and these are all put together in a box; each person has to see if they can recognise their own lemon just by feel.

Self-disclosure

True–false – each person makes (or prepares) three statements about themselves (two true, one false) and the rest of the group has to decide which is the false statement. Alternatively, each person writes a true statement about themselves, puts these in a hat; statements are drawn out and the group has to decide who made it.
Links – love–hate. Each person is given a numbered card at random with something like 'Royal family', 'shoulder pads' written on it. Each topic is taken in turn and the group string themselves along an imaginary line as to whether they love, loathe or feel indifferent (middle of line).
Household object – each person describes a household object (kettle, double bed, coffee table) which they feel reflects their present mood, how they see themselves, etc. This can be done using animals rather than objects.
Objects in the bag – participants take two or three objects out of their bag/pockets and other group members have to make a story/picture of the person from these objects.

Looking specifically at power and oppression

(though note that all these games have a power dimension)
Stereotyping – in pairs, participants deliberately make assumptions about their partner (which newspaper they read, etc.) and share these assumptions.
Power cards – participants take a collection of card descriptions which apply to them (e.g. woman; white; professional, etc.) and decide how much power (in a scale of one to ten, least to most powerful) they feel each one ascribes them; these can be shared with a partner or the whole group, looking at different situations to see if this changes how they view the power balance.

Closure

Feedback on the back – each person has a piece of paper pinned to their back and other group members write positive statements about them on the paper for them to take away with them.

Fit kit

There is much to learn from the groupwork portfolios (see Chapter 1) about the use of 'kit' in groups, especially the use of video, whether pre-recorded or recording live. Video as a piece of kit in groups drew a wide range of comments. For example:

> The evaluation feedback suggests that using [video] clips sparingly was the most successful approach.
>
> Portfolio P, 4.2

> [With the benefit of experience] we now introduce the video camera from day one and record every session, so its introduction is less dramatic and people get used to it very quickly.
>
> Portfolio C, 2.1

The specificity of video, cultural and otherwise, suggests caution in the way it is used. Indeed, with any groupwork method or technique, the first and last question is, *how is it fit for purpose?* This should prevent you extracting an activity from your tool kit just to fill a gap.

Increasing your range of methods and techniques should mean that you are able to diversify your groupwork and respond more sensitively to needs in the group. If all you have is a 'hammer', you will find it difficult to help the group 'fix a screw'. Using a discerning variety of methods is more likely to charge the group's energy levels; it also recognises that people have different responses.

> The relaxation and meditation techniques didn't suit some members of the group because they couldn't concentrate or keep the focus, whilst others really enjoyed the exercise.
>
> Portfolio H, 4.2

BOX 5.7 USING A RANGE OF METHODS

Offending Awareness group – session on victim awareness

1 *What is a victim?* Group brainstorm using the whiteboard to come up with an agreed definition of 'a victim'.
2 *How do people become victims?* Group members asked to decide under what circumstances people become victims (e.g. natural disasters, bullying, crime, etc.)

break for refreshments

3 *The 'deserving' victim.* Prior to the session, three large cards with the words *To Blame, Don't Know* and *Not To Blame* had been placed on three separate walls

Box 5.7 continued

in the room. I explained to the group that they would hear a selection of crime/ victim scenarios and for each they must decide which card on the wall they most agreed with and stand next to it. I then encouraged group members to discuss their choice and reasons for their answer.

4   *Is it fair?* Game in which cards with statistics are placed alongside cards with statements on a table in the middle of the room. Young people are asked to work together as a group to match up the correct figure with its accompanying statement. We then discussed as a group if this seemed right/fair and reasons for our responses.

break

5   *Hidden victims/victimless crimes.* Each young person was given a crime scenario from a pre-prepared list, for example:

   a) the broken glass and hanging around in the park
   b) stealing the can of coke
   c) vandalising the phone box

The group members watched a short video regarding victims of crime with their scenario in mind and wrote down the following (displayed on a flipchart throughout the video playing):

   a) who is affected/who are the victims?
   b) how are they affected?
   c) how might they feel?

We then shared and discussed each individual's answers as a group.

6   *Closing summary.* Asked members to look again at the aims of the session written on flipchart paper at the beginning and to see if they could tell me which exercise met which aim.

7   *Goodbyes* and reminders of the next session, and travel fares distributed.

Portfolio O, 3.3.

Ultimately, the decision about which methods to use and when, should be guided by the central notion of group purpose. As we learned in Chapter 4, purpose is not confined to outcomes (♠). A wider sense of purpose must encompass feelings (♥), processes (♦) and contexts (♣), and the methods used in any one session should cover all four suits.

ACTIVITY 5.5: FIT FOR PURPOSE

It is important to consider each activity carefully. How does it meet this group's particular purposes at this particular time? Check, for example, that an ice-breaker hasn't become just habitual or a personal favourite of one of the group leaders!

Consider the ice-breakers, warm-ups and cool-downs in Box 5.6, and the activities in Box 5.7.

Which kinds of purpose might each of these different activities fulfil for the group? From this, you should develop criteria which you could use to help you consider what kind of activity to introduce into the group and when.

(An example response is given in the Appendix.)

Groupworkers should work towards the group itself taking increasing control, as the group learns more about methods and techniques and their use.

> Some didn't like certain background music and we changed this frequently. We reached common ground in the end by using visualisation techniques. The group was assertive in that if they did not approve of some techniques they would express their views to us.
>
> Portfolio H, 6.2

The Westville Women's group used a method which was already familiar (the Links game) to help the group make priorities about future activities (Box 5.5). With growing knowledge and confidence, group members can start to construct their own sessions using methods they have learned through participation in the group. The Links activity also demonstrates the generic nature of so many of the techniques and methods of groupwork. Though the topics in the Links activity will vary from group to group and session to session, the method itself was appropriate to all 54 of the groups in the Groupwork Project (Box 1.1). Indeed, most groupwork methods can readily be used across a broad range of group settings.

KEY POINTS

- Groupwork has an element of performance and each group session requires some 'staging'.
- Improvisation is an essential ingredient of successful groupwork.
- Groups have 'sub-texts' or themes which groupworkers should help the group to articulate – this assists the development of group identity.
- The group's rhythm can be altered by establishing and breaking patterns in the group's sessions.
- It is important to develop a range of different methods and techniques, but to use these fittingly.
- Groupwork is a qualitatively different experience from individual work, largely because of the opportunity for creative playfulness.

FURTHER READING

Doel, M. and Sawdon, C. (1999), *The Essential Groupworker: Teaching and Learning Creative Groupwork,* London: Jessica Kingsley.
    Chapter 6 presents a wide range of 'action techniques' for groupworkers to use with groups.
Fuchs, B. (2002), *Group Games: Social Skills,* Bicester: Speechmark.
    This book contains 160 practical ideas to improve the social climate within groups of people and can be used with a wide variety of groups and teams.
Groupwork journal (London: Whiting and Birch, issues from 1989–present) provides a rich variety of examples of groups in action.

LEAD?

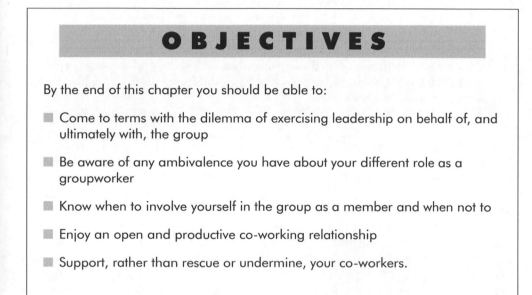

OBJECTIVES

By the end of this chapter you should be able to:

- Come to terms with the dilemma of exercising leadership on behalf of, and ultimately with, the group

- Be aware of any ambivalence you have about your different role as a groupworker

- Know when to involve yourself in the group as a member and when not to

- Enjoy an open and productive co-working relationship

- Support, rather than rescue or undermine, your co-workers.

LEADERS AND MEMBERS

> Two anxieties expressed by social workers leading groups are, paradoxically, discomfort about authority and the fear of losing control.
>
> (Brown, 1994: 74)

Power, authority and control

When groupworkers put their cards on the table at the beginning of the first session (see Chapter 4), one of the profound differences between members and workers in the group is made transparent: the group leaders are seldom in the same boat as the group members (though see Maram and Rice, 2002; Mistry and Brown, 1997). Choice of pronoun soon highlights this. It may be 'we' who will be working together, but it is 'you' who are experiencing the difficulties. Mandy recognised this distinction in the group where members are foster carers and the workers are social care workers:

> In our 'Cards on the Table' we tried to emphasize that WE weren't the experts and that the group members' experience with foster children was far more important and valid in terms of sharing information and knowledge. Yet, I feel that they did see us as having power, through position and knowledge; we had, after all, set the aims and objectives as well as the structure of the group before it had even begun.
>
> Portfolio M, 2.P&O

Again, Mandy underlines the discomfort many groupworkers feel about handling the fact that they are in different circumstances to group members.

> We wanted to reassure the group members that we understood, to some degree, how they felt, but that in fact we had no experience as foster carers. Having said that, we needed to realize that the tactics and strategies we would be talking about were applicable to all children and therefore just as useful to them as foster carers.
>
> Portfolio M, 2.3

Much will depend on the genesis of the group. In groups that are already firmly in the hands of the membership, such as many social action groups, practitioners might already be playing supporting roles (Mullender and Ward, 1991), perhaps more as consultants. As Constable and Frysztacki (1994: 32) note, 'a good consultant ... is really a catalyst for already existing possibilities'.

For those groups where the workers have been instrumental in its creation, recruiting the membership and making the arrangements, the leadership which is implicit in these activities cannot suddenly be abandoned. The paradox is that the groupworkers must exercise leadership in order to transfer it to the group membership, hence the question mark in this chapter's title. Indeed, learning about positive leadership from the groupworkers can be a significant outcome for the group. A group where leadership is not exercised can find itself dominated by the most powerful individuals within the group; in other words, it will merely mimic the processes of discrimination and oppression which take place in the wider community. If the group as a whole is to be empowered, rather than its most powerful individuals, it will need to learn to behave counter-culturally; in other words, in ways which are not prevalent in the wider world outside the group. Social groupworkers have a powerful role to play in developing anti-oppressive and anti-discriminatory values and behaviours in the group.

Groups which are heavily scripted with full programmes devised by the group leaders (or external experts), with purposes strongly oriented towards outcomes and product, must beware the steamroller effect. In these circumstances, how can the leaders' authority be used to empower the group as a whole? For example, the script must allow time for the group to negotiate its own ground rules, with proper attention to how it can influence and change the course of the script itself. Even apparently small details have a significance for the message which the groupworkers are communicating about their leadership style.

I would perhaps change the layout of the room so that Meg [co-worker] and I had been more a 'part' of the group, rather than appearing to be at the 'head' of it.

Portfolio M, 2.3

Part of the exercise of leadership is the exercise of control. Because of the pejorative connotations of words like 'controlling', groupworkers sometimes shy away from control, yet it is of fundamental value in groups. Ironically, fear of losing it is possibly one of the main reasons why many do not practise groupwork. Group members will not attend a group they feel is out of control, since it will be perceived as unsafe, but exercising control in ways which are experienced as empowering demands skill. At all times, you should think of yourself as exercising control *on behalf of the group*, until such time that the group can fairly exercise this control itself.

Sometimes the groupworker's power is best exercised outside the full glare of the group, though this does deny the group as a whole the opportunity to learn more about how power, authority and control can be fairly exercised in the group.

After the second session of the group I spoke to Simon on his own when we were making coffee. I explained to him that his behaviour was making it difficult for the group and Sonia [my co-worker] and me. He said he was having a hyper day and that it was just him. I said this was unreasonable which he agreed with and he said he would try to calm down and stop interrupting. I thanked him. Simon's behaviour hindered the group and on the two occasions he did not attend, the rest of the group were relaxed and happy to speak aloud.

Portfolio S, 5.1

ACTIVITY 6.1: EXERCISING CONTROL ON BEHALF OF THE GROUP

Sound Start group

Simon, a sixteen-year old, constantly interrupted or played with his phone. He deliberately changed the subject and asked unrelated questions. Simon did this because he was 'having a hyper day'.

- What would you do?

You now have the following information about Simon:

Simon was a very powerful person in the group, the only male. He enjoyed this and sought to strengthen his position each session by being the centre of attention and by taking control of conversations. Simon also fancied Stacey [another group member] and was trying to seek her approval by being funny. This situation was 'named' at times, particularly when it broke the group agreement, such as interrupting, sexist jokes, using mobile phone, being unhelpful. Simon apologised each time, but after several minutes it started again.

Portfolio S, 5.1

- What would you have done?

As well as exercising control on behalf of the group, groupworkers hold considerable power in their ability to reward. There is implied reward in the attention of the 'group's gaze', but everyone in the group has opportunity to give more explicit rewards, in the form of positive feedback. Workers will probably have to model rewarding before group members feel comfortable to use it, especially since the dominant British culture is sparing with this kind of reward, and it is readily seen as patronising or manipulative. Care should be taken about how rewards are used; for example, remembering to reward the group as a whole, to reinforce group identity.

ACTIVITY 6.2: THE POWER OF REWARD

Sound Start group

> I was very proud of Sharleen, given her learning difficulties and how difficult she had found it to attend the first session, and this was 'named' outside the group setting and sometimes during the session. When Sharleen was working hard I would name it by saying something like, 'Sharleen seems to be doing a good job on her handout. That's really good.'
>
> Portfolio S, 5.1

- What are the benefits of rewarding Sharleen in this way?
- What are potential risks of this?
- How might this reward be complemented with a reward for the group as a whole?

(An example response is given in the Appendix.)

Physical control is not an uncommon issue for groups involving young people, and the narrative in Box 6.1 (from the portfolio of Orla's co-worker, Oliver) indicates how rapidly a situation can move out of control and, indeed, how quickly the skilled groupworker can bring it back. This kind of incident tends to be the groupworker's bad fantasy; however, it is actually the group where there is a slow drift away from purpose that is the more challenging, since it is not so obvious that this group is in crisis.

Ambivalence and difference

If social workers feel ambivalent about exercising authority in work with individuals, they are likely to feel it even more so with groups (Reid, 1988). The motivation for social work is more usually about helping than exercising control, and the analysis of social structures focuses on oppressive and unjust uses of power. Groupworkers are often acutely aware of the fact that they are not in the same boat as the group members and the lack of experiential authority which this implies. So, it is unsurprising that social groupworkers can feel uncomfortable exercising the authority of leadership in groups.

> ### BOX 6.1 FLARE UP
>
> **Offending Awareness group**
>
> Orla's co-worker, Oliver, notes in his portfolio how he mediated between two group members, Owen and Oz, in a session on anger management.
>
> O'Connor: What would you know, you've never left the estate for more than a day, you and your little gang.
>
> Oz: Says he! You talk about fighting when you've run off before!
>
> O'Connor: Piss off! [stands up]. At least I sort things out myself and don't hide behind my boys!
>
> Oliver: Whoa, whoa, whoa! [gestures for them to sit down] Now, come on lads! I think we've gone off the point a little here [they sit down]. Nice as it is to see some real-life anger in the room …
>
> O'Connor: But he started it! I'm trying to tell you about when I can't cope and he butts in. I was talking, not him.
>
> Oliver: Yeh, and you've worked well together up to now. It doesn't matter what happened in the past, I don't expect you to be best mates, but for one thing it does show you how anger can be sudden and soon get out of control.
>
> Portfolio O1, 5.2

Nevertheless, it is important that ambivalence does not inhibit groupworkers from using the authority of their position in the group when the group needs it. Fran, a groupworker in the Family Support group (Box 1.F) heard some of the members making critical remarks about the African and Asian themed days which the group held during the summer holidays. Fran, who is dual heritage, reflected in her portfolio on the processes which finally led her to overcome her doubts and to exercise her authority in the group, with beneficial results. (See Box 7.3 for more details about this situation.)

> I am aware that the criticisms and racism in the weeks that followed had an impact on how I felt about and worked with these group members. I realized that I had internalized many of the comments as I have a very strong dislike of racism since I have been and am subjected to it. Filomena [a black co-worker] did not 'see' the racist connotations, so I discussed my feelings with a black ex-colleague and friend and decided that in order to move on I had to discuss this with the people involved. Having done this, I have found that it has not only helped us to move forward [in the group], but has gone some ways to improving our relationships, the people in question are no longer afraid to ask questions about my heritage.
>
> Portfolio F, 4.1

Ambivalence is often rooted in our feelings about difference, and this sense of difference can be perceived in various ways. The obvious differences, such as race, may or may not be the ones which become significant in the group, and differences may be felt not just between groupworkers and members, but also amongst the members themselves.

> Winsome [one of the group members] owns her own house, which gives her a certain prestige in the eyes of the other group members. The women also view me and Win [co-worker] as well-off because we have cars.
>
> Portfolio W, 4.P&O

The group has a choice about whether and how to address difference. Accepting and respecting difference can be core to the achievement of group identity – an identity which is often at odds with the social norms outside the group. Indeed, the group's *difference* from the world outside can be an illuminating way for the group to work with its own internal differences.

BOX 6.2 LEADER-MEMBER DIFFERENCES

Sound Start group

Samantha makes the differences between her own circumstances and those of the group members starkly clear.

> My own biography is almost at the other end of the spectrum from that of the group members. I was brought up in a stable and loving family where I lived until I was 18 when I left home and went to university. I have had a good education and I work full-time. I have stable friends and family. I have no personal experience of being rejected by my family, living with a variety of strangers, having professional people plan my life, and having little control over any aspect of my life. I have not had my life messed about by inconsistent adults who do not always have my best interests at heart.
>
> Portfolio S, 8.1

ACTIVITY 6.3: WORKING WITH DIFFERENCE

Sound Start group
What positive and negative impact might the differences described by Samantha in Box 6.2 have on her leadership of the group?

Participation

Groupworkers have choices about their role in the group's activities. For example, when there is 'a round' and individuals in the group are invited to give an example of their own experience, should groupworkers contribute their own experience? Often they do not have the direct experience in question (for example, attempting suicide), and to talk about the experiences of other people they have worked with or known would be inappropriate. However, a round which focused on 'what we expect from this group' would be one in which the groupworkers could be expected to participate.

So, the groupworker is both a leader and a member of the group. Managing these seemingly contradictory roles is a key aspect of successful groupworking, made concrete when deciding when to participate *as a group member.* When playing a game such as 'Links' (Box 5.5), do the groupworkers place themselves along the imaginary line as part of the group's links? Working on Activity 6.4 will help you (and any co-worker) to consider why and when you would choose to join in or opt out.

ACTIVITY 6.4: JOINING IN

Return to the eight ways to develop group identity in Box 5.3. In which of these eight activities would you expect to participate alongside group members, and which not? What have you based your decisions on? Thinking of the nine groups which illustrate this book, how might the different memberships of these groups affect your decision about joining in?

As a rule of thumb, it is more appropriate for groupworkers to participate as group members when the focus is on the group *as a group.* Although the groupworkers have a different role in the group, they are nevertheless *in* the group. Of course, there is no clear line of definition, and even when groupworkers do participate appropriately, they need to be aware that this will usually be seen as being on different terms. Indeed, group members might quite literally see the groupworker differently. Paul, watching the video made of the last session of the Parenting Skills group, notes that Penny 'misinterprets some of my non-verbal communication: "you're frowning" ' (Portfolio P, 9.1). Where Paul sees concern, Penny sees disapproval.

The observer of Wendy's groupwork practice noted the co-workers' participation positively, but you will see in Activity 6.5 that Wendy herself records a dilemma as a result of joining in an activity.

> Wendy and Win [the co-workers] joined in all the exercises, which I felt made the exercises seem less threatening, and they shared some of their experiences and feelings.
>
> Portfolio W, 9.2

ACTIVITY 6.5: FOLLOW MY LEADER

Westville Women's group
The group are doing the Links activity (details in Box 5.5). You note the following developments:

> It was unusual for the group members to experience us, the groupworkers, joining in the same activity. As a result they may have copied us, assuming it may be the 'right' answer. One of the topics on the cards was PUBLIC TRANSPORT. Along with Win, my co-worker, I placed myself at the 'like' end of the Link, and was followed by all the other group members. But I knew that Winsome did not like travelling on public transport at all, because she had previously told me so.
>
> (adapted from Portfolio W, 6.P&O)

• What do you do?

The groupworker role provides a different experience to the one which the worker experiences in much of their work as a social worker, occupational therapist, health visitor, and the like. Fran notes this explicitly in her work with the Family Support group.

> Group members sometimes 'forget' our roles as social workers.
> Portfolio F, 2.1

There is some evidence from the Groupwork Project (Box 1.1) that part of the attraction of groupwork is, indeed, the permission to step into a different role. So, it is not just group members, but the groupworkers, too, who might forget that they are social workers. Perhaps those colleagues who are less than supportive to groupwork are, in fact, hankering after a similar kind of change. They intuit that, when their colleagues become groupworkers 'they change their clothes'.

Participation in activities such as Links (Box 5.5) leads to much more self-disclosure by the worker than is likely in individual contact. Indeed, intimacy is a key factor in groupwork. Knowing how to wear the cloak of authority and when to take it off is as much art as science.

> This Crimestop programme places emphasis on group leaders sharing more than is normally the case. Giving (appropriately) something of ourselves to the group is advocated from the start. However, each leader has to decide what this means for themselves.
> Portfolio C, 4.P&O

The difference, and potential conflict, between the role inside and outside the group can be highlighted when the groupworker is also the individual worker for some of the members in the group, as Helen notes with the Women of Hope group (Box 1.H).

It was difficult for me when we got into sticky situations [in the group], because they tended to expect different approaches from me, the fact that I was their worker in individual sessions ... I would prefer in the future to do groupwork with people for whom I don't do individual work ... At times, when I visited them individually at home, they wanted to discuss group issues.

Portfolio H, 3.1

Members leading

References to 'the group' suggest an altogether more coherent entity than in most realities. The group consists of a complex and changing set of dynamics between individuals and subgroups; whereas the sense of self is continuous, the sense of group is temporary. Even in groups with a strong sense of identity, individual behaviours and roles are likely to differ considerably. In this context, we can see how the injunction to 'empower the group' is easier written than done. In sloughing off their power (to the extent that this is possible and desirable), the groupworkers may find that it is individual group members who take up the mantle rather than 'the group'.

Is this a problem? Empowering certain individuals at the expense of others would not be true to anti-oppressive principles, and other group members might find it more acceptable for the groupworkers to exercise leadership rather than fellow members. However, if one or more group members can provide leadership which is inclusive and not exclusive, which is respectful of the group as a whole, and which continues to attempt to broaden leadership and authority within the group, we can see this as a success. It is an important step towards the group becoming self-running if this is how the group wants to move. It is a mistake for groupworkers to perceive the development of this style of 'internal leadership' as a threat to their own control; if it does pose a threat, it is to the integrity of the group as a whole.

The dynamic of power in the group is highly complex, as both Samantha and Claire both note in different contexts:

Stacey became powerful by choosing to be powerless. In being silent she had manipulated the whole group into focusing on her and whatever her problems were. Stacey has learning difficulties and I feel that she has learned behaviours which get her attention and give her the power that her learning difficulties take away. This can be seen as both manipulative and resourceful, depending on her motive.

Portfolio S, 8.1

A sub-group of entrenched drug users often colluded with one another, having its own leader. When that leader has been away, another quieter group member spoke more freely and 'from the heart'.

Portfolio C, 5.P&O

One of the groupworker's tasks is to find ways to help the group to become aware of power, authority and control in the group, so that the group as a whole can develop reference points and language to recognise abuses and to challenge them, whether these emanate from other group members or from the groupworkers themselves.

CO-WORKING

All told, 68 groups were planned as a result of the Groupwork Project and 54 successfully ran their course (details in Box 1.1). Of these, almost nine out of ten were co-led, in most cases by two groupworkers ($n = 47$; 87%). This is not a surprising statistic given that groupwork learners were strongly encouraged to apply to the project in pairs and to co-work. More illuminating is the fact that of the 14 groups which were planned and did not materialise, 5 involved single-worker groups. The percentage of single-led groups in the failed sample (36%) is, therefore, much higher than the percentage of single-led groups in the successful sample ($n = 7$; 13%). What are the benefits, then, of co-working?

Co-working as a model for group members

> Most of the potential benefits for group members arise from having two workers with distinctive characteristics who, in combination, can offer the group and individual member more than either would be able to alone.
>
> Brown (1994: 78)

Brown's assertion above is the accepted wisdom of co-working in groups. There was some support for this view within the experience of the project, for example in Orla's accounts of the mixed gender co-leadership of the Offending Awareness group. Paul, too, appreciated the significance of his co-working with Petra in the Parents Plus group.

> Our co-leader gender balance was able to model a more respectful and open way [than the women in the group had experienced].
>
> Portfolio P, 5.P&O

However, more commonly, workers were drawn to co-work with others who had similar, rather than different, characteristics. Of the 47 co-led groups, almost three out of five were co-led by two or more white women ($n = 27$; 57%). A bruising session with a male co-worker, Steve, led Samantha to conclude that 'the group benefited more by having co-workers *with a good relationship*, which I found working with Sonia' (Portfolio S, 2.2 – my emphasis). Samantha felt that the sessions when she co-worked with Sonia were the best.

Only two of the groups had a mixed race co-leadership, one of which was the Family Support group. This was also one of the few groups in which ethnicity and race were made explicit topics within the group itself (see Box 7.3).

> On the Asian and African days, the co-workers organised specific events to relate to these themes, which included music, food, photographs, arts and dress. Filomena led the preparations for the African theme day ... and I led the Asian theme day.
>
> Portfolio F, 2.2

It seems likely that, in practice, co-working is motivated less by a desire for diversity and more for mutual support.

Multiple co-workers

Anecdotal evidence suggests that there is an increase in multiple co-working, of which there are two kinds. The first is a regular group of three or more co-workers who work together most of the time. This is often the response when there are additional demands on groupworkers' time and resources, such as the Memory Joggers group (Box 1.J). The second model of multiple groupworking is when there are three or more co-workers involved, but only two of them are co-working in any particular session. Sometimes there might be a lead worker who is always present for continuity purposes, such as Samantha with the Sound Start group. Involving most of the team in this way can increase support for the group. The whole of Orla's team was involved in the Offending Awareness group, with different people responsible for the planning and co-working for particular sessions; for example, Orla was responsible for the lead on the victim awareness sessions.

An arrangement of multiple groupworkers can be beneficial in a number of ways. On a practical level, it spreads the load of preparing and facilitating groups, and ensures the group is sufficiently resourced to withstand absences by groupworkers.

> Additional benefits include cover if one co-worker is on holiday, has other commitments that can't be avoided or is absent. On no occasion has the group been unable to run, which is an achievement. When all co-workers are present we are able to offer a wider variety of choice to group members.
>
> Portfolio J, 2.2

Jenny and her three co-facilitators had planned the group together, working closely as members of the same team and making time to review the group's progress. In contrast to Jenny, Claire's experience tended to confirm Brown's (1994) caution about the confusion about roles which multiple leadership models can cause. Claire was part of a large team of groupworkers, but one which had no regular pattern of commitment or contact with the group, or communication with one another.

> I would change the way a number of group leaders dip in and out over the length of the programme. This has been incredibly disruptive and various groups have responded differently. Some have become withdrawn, others aggressive.
>
> Portfolio C, 5.3

It is important that group members are not overwhelmed by a leadership of three or more groupworkers. Communication between co-workers can be complex, and some co-workers may find it hard to keep 'up to speed'. Orla and her team colleagues worked hard to research their particular topics for the Offending Awareness group. The support workers were involved in the group but not in the research for the topics. 'One of the support workers explained how he felt that he had to work harder to gain a clear understanding of aims and purposes of each session due to his lack of direct involvement from the start' (Portfolio O, 2.2).

Even in the smooth-running multiple leadership of the Memory Joggers group, it was well into the life of the group before Jenny came to realise that one of her co-workers, Joy, a social care worker, had a very different conception of the group to her own. This transpired during one of the groupwork training sessions.

> It did surprise me that Joy was of the impression that the group was only a social gathering. I had assumed otherwise.
>
> Portfolio J, 2.2

Support and rescue

Co-workers are important sources of support for one another. Both outside and inside the group they should provide feedback about their individual and joint performance and, when the co-working is sound, they are a safety net for one another.

> Before the session we had discussed thoroughly how we would deal with incidents and potential problems. This feeling of certain support from my co-leader helped to reassure me during my worst moments of panic before beginning the session.
>
> Portfolio O, 3.2

Leading or facilitating a group is demanding work, especially attending to the needs of the group as a whole at the same time as to the needs of individual members. Between them, co-workers can cover both of these bases. For example, in Activity 6.2 we saw that Samantha was rewarding an individual group member. At the same time her co-worker could pick up on the possible effect on the group as a whole and look for an opportunity to reward the group, too. Co-workers can rescue failed explanations or interventions by their partner, though it is always important, following the group session, to talk through the partner's feelings about the rescue – supportive or undermining?

> On one occasion I introduced an exercise and did it in a lacklustre way. It was a *desert island* exercise whereby the group must make a list of rules to live by on a desert island. Chris [my co-worker] came in and added to the explanation in a tactful way to inject a little more enthusiasm. On another occasion he reminded me to tell the group why we were doing a particular exercise to make it relevant to them. Both these contributions by Chris were helpful.
>
> Portfolio C, 5.3

ACTIVITY 6.6: RESCUE OR SUPPORT?

Offending Awareness group
Given the situation in Box 6.3, what would you do or say? What would you expect your co-worker to do or say?

BOX 6.3 CO-WORKING WHEN IT'S DIFFICULT

Offending Awareness group

Orla is co-leading the Offending Awareness group with boys aged 14 to 17 years old who are attending the group by order of the court.

In one particular session covering issues surrounding sexual health and teenage pregnancy, all but one of the group members continually tried to draw Orla's male co-worker into the role of being 'one of the lads' and made inappropriate or prejudicial comments about women throughout the first half of the session, for example, upon providing statistics concerning both men and women and contraction of sexual diseases:

Co-worker: In the Oldtown area alone, 75% of women tested at GUM [genito-urinary medical] clinics have been diagnosed as having some kind of sexually transmitted infection, and 62% of men.

O'Connor: That's because most girls in Oldtown are slappers and will sleep with anyone!

Portfolio O, 2.2

Competition and other difficulties

Although co-working is a popular arrangement, it is not without its difficulties. In response to the question, *What were your feelings and thoughts before the first session of the group?*, three of Helen's five concerns related to the co-working situation. In particular, she wrote of her concerns about her own competence, especially in front of her co-worker, perhaps heightened by the fact that the co-worker was from a different professional group (Box 1.H).

What would the co-worker think of my practice and performance on the day?

Portfolio H, 3.2

The experience of co-working may be the first time that your direct practice is witnessed in a systematic way by a colleague. Moreover, there is also the 'comparison effect' – will group members prefer my co-worker? As Orla prepared to lead the first session of her block on victim awareness, she describes her apprehensions:

Some of the young people had already participated in sessions led by my colleagues, and a key factor in my apprehension was pressure, albeit self-inflicted, about whether my session would be enjoyed as much as previous sessions, and run as smoothly.

Portfolio O, 3.2

Co-workers with very different styles will need to agree a *modus operandi* with which they are both happy. The first step is to be aware of these differences, as Samantha notes below. However, as we shall see in the next chapter, awareness of different styles is not enough to prevent difficulties in the group.

> Steve and I are used to working together but have very different ways of working. Steve is laid back and happier to take things as they come. I am the opposite and like to have everything organised in advance.
>
> Portfolio S, 1.1

There are many ways in which co-workers can ensure that they and the group find this a mutually beneficial relationship (see Box 6.4). In particular, you must ensure that you spend time working through any differences. Regular reviews should enable frank exchanges of view about each other's work and give expression to group members' views on the leadership. As one of the members of the Parents Plus group noted on her evaluation sheet:

> Great double act! (Portfolio P, Appendix)

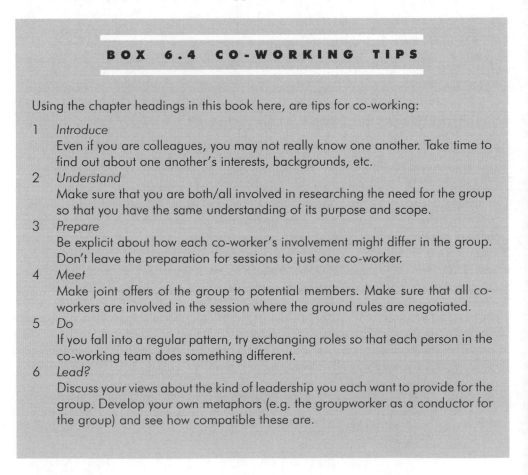

BOX 6.4   CO-WORKING   TIPS

Using the chapter headings in this book here, are tips for co-working:

1   *Introduce*
    Even if you are colleagues, you may not really know one another. Take time to find out about one another's interests, backgrounds, etc.
2   *Understand*
    Make sure that you are both/all involved in researching the need for the group so that you have the same understanding of its purpose and scope.
3   *Prepare*
    Be explicit about how each co-worker's involvement might differ in the group. Don't leave the preparation for sessions to just one co-worker.
4   *Meet*
    Make joint offers of the group to potential members. Make sure that all co-workers are involved in the session where the ground rules are negotiated.
5   *Do*
    If you fall into a regular pattern, try exchanging roles so that each person in the co-working team does something different.
6   *Lead?*
    Discuss your views about the kind of leadership you each want to provide for the group. Develop your own metaphors (e.g. the groupworker as a conductor for the group) and see how compatible these are.

> **Box 6.4 continued**
>
> 7 *Beware*
> Use a sentence-completion exercise of potentially difficult situations; look at how your responses differ and decide what you would do about these differences (Doel and Sawdon, 1999a: 214–16).
> 8 *Value*
> Hold regular reviews to develop honest communication; in all the practicalities of groupwork, don't lose the values that underpin it.
> 9 *Grow*
> See if you can undertake continuing professional development together; the focus need not be on groupwork itself. Give access to one another's portfolios or professional accounts of learning from the group experience.

KEY POINTS

- Everyone in a group is a member of that group, including the groupworkers.
- However, groupworkers have a different role in the group, and this difference can be difficult to handle.
- Groupworkers should embrace the authority of their leadership role, but they should exercise leadership on behalf of the group, encouraging the group to assume this role as appropriate.
- Co-working is a very common arrangement but it needs careful maintenance to ensure that the co-workers and the group as a whole get the most benefit from it.

FURTHER READING

Lee, F.W. and Yim, E.L. (2004) 'Experiential learning group for leadership development of young people', *Groupwork,* 14.3, pp. 63–90, London: Whiting and Birch.
This article takes up one of the themes in this chapter, that group members can learn about leadership through their experiences of groupwork.

Mistry, T. and Brown, A. (eds) (1997) *Race and Groupwork,* London: Whiting and Birch.
This book takes up the themes of inclusion and exclusion, similarity and difference, with specific reference to race and groupwork.

Mullender, A. and Ward, D. (1991) *Self-Directed Groupwork: Users Take Action for Empowerment,* London: Whiting and Birch.
A model of groupwork based on empowerment in which the group takes over by taking action.

CHAPTER 7

BEWARE

OBJECTIVES

By the end of this chapter you should be able to:

■ Identify pitfalls in groups and be aware of those which you feel you are most likely to experience

■ Understand the inadequacy of responses which attempt to accommodate, compromise or confront

■ Respond to critical incidents and dilemmas as opportunities for group learning

■ Use the 'line of enquiry' approach to work *with* the group rather than against it

■ Enable the group to take increasing responsibility for its own learning.

POTENTIAL PITFALLS

Difficulties in groups and teams are amplified by the complex dynamics involved, and their semi-public nature. This is perhaps why the idea of groups and groupwork can seem intimidating. This chapter confronts some of these bad fantasies about groupwork (not always fantasies), as evidenced from the Groupwork Project (Box 1.1). I will use the four 'suits' which were introduced in Chapter 4 to consider what we need to beware in groupwork practice.

♠ Outcomes

Over-programming

> Craig accused the group leaders of not caring for the group. He said he felt
> we should have an informal chat at the start of each group to address any
> issues individuals had concerns about. I believe that Craig had issues he
> wanted to talk to the group about and felt the need for some open space
> within which to do this. This is not catered for in this [Crimestop] programme
> … His needs conflicted with the needs of the group.
>
> Portfolio C, 2.1

… or did Craig's needs conflict with those of the programme rather than those of the
group? The drive to achieve successful outcomes, as defined by the group programmers,
can squeeze out any space in the group for unprogrammed discussion and activity.
Over-programming can lead group members to behave as passengers, since the
responsibility for the group is never theirs. Of course, the balance between over-
programming and programme drift is an important one:

> … group members made comments such as 'we only did half of what is on
> the programme'. This tended to happen through poor planning and time
> management within the group session, rather than spontaneous change of
> plans initiated by the group itself … An hour before the group began Steve,
> my co-worker, decided that we could make pancakes with the group and
> that it would fit into the timing of the programme. I strongly disagreed and
> suggested that we would not have time to get through what had been planned,
> or at least we could leave it until the end if we had time. Steve decided to go
> ahead anyway. Understandably, the group thought that making pancakes
> was most enjoyable! However, we only got through half of what was planned
> and the session was disrupted due to the group being excited at the prospect
> of cooking. Few, if any, of the aims were achieved and the session dissolved
> into an eating frenzy.
>
> Portfolio S, 2.2

♥ Feelings

Repressing differences

Just as a social work encounter is different from an everyday conversation, so a group
session is not the same as a social gathering in a group. Social behaviour in groups tends
towards consensus and avoidance of conflict, but the group in the context of social
groupwork needs to look for opportunities in which differences can be safely expressed.
This is often a challenge for novice groupworkers who are keen to have the group 'go
well', because they still see their role in social, rather than groupwork, terms.

The desire for a strong consensus can inhibit individuals from expressing different beliefs or feelings. The Links activity (Box 5.5) is a relatively safe way to introduce the group to differences of opinion, acting as a stepping stone to riskier areas of belief and expression. In the Managing Behaviour for Carers group, Mandy was able to encourage Meera, one of the group members, to express what Meera saw as feelings about her foster son that would have been unacceptable outside the group (see Chapter 5, page 91).

Focusing too heavily on your own feelings and performance

Difficulties in groups can often lead you to become so conscious of yourself that you close down communication with the group. It is vital that you 'step to the side of yourself' in these circumstances in order to stay with the group and the individual members (Doel, 2004).

> My own feelings became paramount in the days prior to me attending the group [as a new co-leader] and therefore I did not spend time on trying to perceive the thoughts and feelings of the group members.
>
> Portfolio F, 3.2

Groupworkers need to keep in touch not just with their own feelings, and not just with those of any particular individual, but with the feelings of the group as a whole.

◆ Processes

Making single-sided judgements

One of the dangers of commonly used labels in groupwork such as 'scapegoat', 'dominant member', 'joker' or 'completer-finisher', 'shaper' and 'implementer' (Belbin, 1993) is their tendency to give us a one-dimensional view of the person to whom they are applied. Life is more complicated, and most people are capable of a variety of behaviours which will fall outside the assigned role, though these other behaviours may be missed precisely because they do not fit 'the Role'. Orla observes this complexity in her pen picture of Oz, a member of the Offending Awareness group; and Petra, co-leader in the Parents Plus group, reflects on two very contrasting sides of group member, Pat:

> [Upon being challenged various times about his attempts to monopolise the group] Oz began scapegoating Owen to assume some form of control within the group. However, Oz also often brought humour in an appropriate manner and could greatly enhance the group atmosphere.
>
> Portfolio O, 5.1

> Pat was the most enthusiastic group member. She took on new ideas and tried them out at home. Pat was open to new ideas and converted her old style of parenting – shouting and hitting – to a new style of negotiation and non-violence. ... Pat showed some interest in engaging with other group

members but struggled to listen to others' problems and views. This led to her dominating some sessions and irritating Penny, in particular, as she was not helping others to problem solve.

Portfolio P1, 5.1

The same behaviour can have different meaning depending on time and place and person, as Jenny perceptively comments:

Like Jean, Jim was a comic, but in a different way. Whereas Jean used her humour to cover her memory deficits, Jim used his to draw a crowd.

Portfolio J, 5.1

Switchboarding

It is common in the early stages of a group for much of the discussion to be routed through the group leaders, so that a statement which would be more appropriately said to a particular group member or the group as a whole is made to the groupworker. If this persists, it is a sign that this is still a collection of individuals rather than a group, and the leaders need to consider how they can switch this pattern. Using some of the group identity activities in Box 5.3 will help.

♣ Contexts

Under-estimating the time needed

Making an accurate estimation of the time needed to lead or co-work a group is one the significant factors in its success. A general rule of thumb is that each hour of contact time in the group requires an hour of preparation and an hour of review and evaluation. In other words, a weekly group which meets for one and a half hours for eight sessions will require about 36 hours of each groupworker's time. This is very approximate, and does not include additional time for groupworkers involved in transporting group members. Colleagues, including managers, need to be convinced that the time is worthwhile, especially when there is some prospect that the time spent in preparation may not lead to the successful birth of a group (a 20% chance in the experience of the Groupwork Project, Box 1.1). Enthusiasm has to be tempered by the possibility that the benefits do not, in fact, justify the time and the risks.

What was problematic is that many people expressed an interest in the group but did not turn up on the day.

Portfolio P1, 2.1

Forgetting colleagues

Two social care workers in the Groupwork Project developed and ran an exceptionally successful women's group in a day centre for people with learning disabilities. One woman whose communication was severely limited began to use the flipchart to express herself to the group, another who generally only spoke in expletives left her swearing behind once she came into the group. The groupworkers themselves grew in confidence and professional self-esteem. An unqualified success – except colleagues became increasingly jealous of this group which met behind the 'do not disturb' sign, and the manager, at first supportive, decided that once this group finished no others would follow. What had been an outstanding experience for the particular members of this group and, indeed, for the social care workers who led it, was seen as a threat by their colleagues. The other users of the day centre felt excluded. Full marks for the group itself, but a blank score sheet for the development of a much-needed groupwork service.

In Chapter 2, I suggested the establishment of a planning group as an opportunity to implicate colleagues and others whose support could be crucial. To consider the group as disconnected from the rest of the work in your team or agency can be a fatal mistake.

Cosiness in the group leadership

The propensity in the Groupwork Project for groupworkers to work with co-leaders who were similar rather than different is probably not unusual (see Chapter 6). This can bring a necessary solidarity, such as might be found in an all-black group membership, but it is also important to beware the risk of cosiness inhibiting self-critical practice or challenge.

> I feel that to have had a male social worker may have encouraged a greater response from male single parents and the partners of the female group members.
>
> Portfolio F, 2.2

Neglecting links to the world outside the group

The group's comfort zone can be so successful that it is tempted to forget what lies beyond. Of course, the cocoon-like nature of some groups is central to their purpose, but you should always find opportunities to help the group connect with the outside. Alternatively, the experience of the group might have been especially challenging compared with the day-to-day lives of its members. In either case, groupworkers should consider how to develop an active trade between here-in-the-group and there-in-the-world. Helen recognised this in the Women of Hope group, and made a positive feature of what could have been a difficult transition from group to world:

> You will probably feel very tired and drained today or tomorrow, and this is a normal reaction following these group sessions because you have had to make the effort to get here, you have worked hard in the group and you have released a lot about yourselves and this is challenging.
> *[Following this, the groupworkers would lead the group in a relaxation exercise to conclude the session.]*
>
> Portfolio H, 6.2

ACTIVITY 7.1: SELF AUDIT

Having read the potential pitfalls above, make a list of the three which you think you will need to be most wary about.

- Why these three?
- Are there any others which are not included here, but which you have anticipated?
- How will you avoid these pitfalls?

CRITICAL INCIDENTS AND DILEMMAS

Groups will undoubtedly experience difficult situations. These are sometimes referred to as critical incidents and it is crucial not to lose their value, for it is at these times that the group can learn much about itself (Fatout, 1998; Henchman and Walton, 1993). Groupworkers, too, can gain much from these incidents, since they often create a dilemma which the rest of the group looks to the groupworkers to resolve. This creates its own dilemma, as we will see later.

We will consider some of the more common kinds of dilemma which arise in groups, using examples taken directly from the groups used to illustrate this book.

BOX 7.1 SEVEN CRITICAL INCIDENTS

1 ACCOMMODATION

In reacting to Frank's dominant behaviour, I am reluctant to 'name' it as I feel this could do more harm than good. Despite his abrupt mannerisms, Frank tries to be helpful and is enthusiastic about any projects we undertake as a group … On one specific occasion he ordered Fliss to 'go and put the kettle on, since you've done nothing since you got here'. I felt embarrassed and angry by this statement and I think Fliss did too. I would have liked to openly confront that statement by asking Frank if he felt he could justify what he had just said to Fliss and to inform him how belittled he made her feel by it. But I didn't, and in some senses I feel that I may have condoned the behaviour by not saying anything. In another sense I did not want to 'pull rank' and openly oppress Frank.

Portfolio F, 5.1

2 COMPROMISE

[The group agreed to organise a Christmas fair to raise funds. A relatively new member to the group,] Francine discussed a stall with cross-stitch items that she would make and what we could charge for these items. Another group member agreed that it was a good idea, but felt that her pricing was unrealistic (too expensive). Francine immediately took offence at this comment and started to

---

Box 7.1 continued

argue her point, that the materials for this *were* expensive. In order to reach a happy medium and prevent confrontation I suggested we could look at Francine doing smaller and less expensive items for the stall. At the time this seemed agreeable with the group, or at least it calmed the situation, but Francine refused to attend any further group sessions.

Portfolio F, 6.2

3 CONFRONTATION

Racist jokes are forms of discrimination that are disguised as humour. Anyone challenging them can be seen as spoiling the fun rather than someone addressing racism. On this occasion Ceiron was telling a racist joke and in my challenging him (too directly for this stage of the programme, I now consider) I was seen as being a spoilsport. The discussion then became a one-on-one argument and I allowed him to escalate to the point where he could not risk backing down without losing face, so he continued to become more outrageous.

Portfolio C, 7

4 AN ASIDE

Wanda had previously been homeless and local people knew her by sight as someone who walked the streets. Behind Wanda's back, Wilma had said 'she used to be a dirty tramp, she shouldn't be here with us'.

Portfolio W, 5.2

5 PANDORA

I suggested that many traumas in our life which we have not managed to negotiate could be a major factor in our current situation. I gave an example as a child if we were abused either physically, sexually or emotionally and we didn't have any help to work through it at the time, that it could have a major impact on us. This led immediately to Hayley becoming upset and appearing angry on leaving the room, muttering something under her breath, and very quickly Hannah got up and left, too.

Portfolio H, 4.3

6 CO-WORKER'S SKILL

On one occasion I felt a memory game wasn't running smoothly, but didn't intervene because I was conscious that it was my 'non-qualified' co-workers who were facilitating. I questioned how my intervention may have been interpreted. I wasn't comfortable with my power position within the group and saw it as a negative thing.

Portfolio J, 5.P&O

7 CO-WORKER'S DECISION

I should have been stronger in voicing my concerns [about my co-worker's changes in plan] but I thought it would be more destructive for the group if there were tensions between the co-workers. *[See the quote from Samantha's portfolio in the section on 'Over-programming' earlier in this chapter.]*

Portfolio S, 2.2

ACTIVITY 7.2: RESPONDING TO A CRITICAL INCIDENT

Review the seven critical incidents in Box 7.1 and choose one of them.

- Consider what you would do immediately following the incident as it is described.
- How would your actions be influenced by different contexts? (You can change the backcloth to the scenario to provide yourself with different contexts.)

Return to this activity when you have completed reading the chapter and reconsider your initial response. How has this been changed by what you have learned?

Accommodation, compromise and confrontation

The first three critical incidents illustrate the great challenge of finding the right kind of intervention for the right occasion. When to accommodate, when to compromise and when to confront?

Much of the dilemma for the groupworker arises from the issues of authority, power and control that we considered in Chapter 6. Fran's account (incident #1) reflects a common inhibition for groupworkers when witnessing questionable behaviour in the group but fearful of using their authority to challenge it. Unfortunately, to do nothing is usually taken not just as accommodating this kind of behaviour, but as approval and collusion. Even subtle non-verbals can be powerfully collusive:

> Collusion is both powerful and oppressive and operates in the most subtle ways; e.g. a smile at a discriminatory joke can indicate agreement and approval.
>
> Portfolio C, 5.P&O

Short-cuts to a compromise are often taken by groupworkers who are uncomfortable with the conflict and wish to enforce a quick peace. However, the compromise too often leaves the whole group dissatisfied, not least because it is enforced by the groupworker, and merely postpones the difficulties which the compromise is supposed to bury. They fester, ready to re-surface as soon as any other disagreements arise. In Box 7.1, incident #2, the 'compromise' actually leads to one member leaving.

Direct confrontations are likely to polarise positions in the group, all too often group-workers against group members. The person who is challenged leaps to their own defence and often calls on the support of other group members; then the groupworker feels the need to enter a defence. Alternatively, the group descends into an aggressive silence, feeling scolded or squashed by the groupworker. There is no specific spot on this continuum which offers a satisfactory solution, and we will learn later how the question *when to accommodate, when to compromise and when to confront?* is misleading.

Taboos and disclosure

The fourth critical incident in Box 7.1, the aside made by Wilma, presents a different kind of dilemma because it is often not intended for the group's hearing. It is unassertively said so that the subject of the statement is unaware of it. Sometimes groupworkers will only be aware of the non-verbal ripples emanating from an aside made by one group member to another, or they may half-hear some of it, uncertain quite what was said and about whom. Certainly, groupworkers cannot let any of this pass by, because this will (rightly) be interpreted as collusive. It needs to be addressed, though there are different ways to do this, as we will see in the section on retrieval strategies.

In helping the group to move beyond its comfort zone, it is inevitable that topics will be introduced which are emotive, even painful. Sometimes the groupworker will be unaware of the resonance of a particular statement, and at other times a calculated risk is taken that opening Pandora's box in a safe environment might encourage the group to face its demons (Box 7.1, incident #5). This might be the first time that someone has been able to speak about a taboo issue, and it will be experienced as a very tense, though possibly cathartic, occasion.

The group should help people to disclose, but this process can be bumpy, with some individual members more willing than others, and some stepping over the invisible boundary of the group's tolerance. The groupworker's intimate knowledge of some of the group members can also create a dilemma about how far to prompt people. For example, at one point in the Crimestop group, Claire thought that Carl's experience as a bus driver would be very relevant to the discussion, but he did not mention it. She did not know whether it was diffidence on his part, whether he genuinely had not made the connection, or whether he was choosing not to let this part of his history be known. This is a situation where the refreshment break is useful, when Claire could ask Carl quietly whether he had thought of mentioning his experience as a bus driver, and she would have got some indication as to whether he would have liked her to have raised it for him.

Groupworkers face decisions about how much of their own lives to disclose. For Claire this was a direct question about whether she was married. Another groupworker described how there were opportunities in the group to discuss sexuality, but acknowledged they 'could not act truthfully' about their own sexuality, based on their experiences of an intolerant society. 'We have assumed that members are heterosexual by the nature and context of their conversation, but this may not necessarily be the case' (Portfolio X). Gay and bisexual groupworkers face these kinds of decision on a daily basis and not just in their groupwork, though groups put them under more of a spotlight.

Co-working dilemmas

In Chapter 6 we learned about co-workers as an important source of support to one another, but also as a possible source of stress. In the last two critical incidents in Box 7.1, there are concerns about the skills of a co-worker (incident #6) and about their judgement (incident #7). The decision to intervene or not when you feel that your co-leader's part of a session is not running well presents an especial dilemma. You do not want to undermine your co-worker's authority, especially if you already suspect they might feel junior to you, and you do not wish to give the group an opportunity to exploit evident differences between you and your co-worker, as was the fear in incident #7. However, to balance this, you are concerned for the quality of the experience of group members and the overall direction of the group. Again, we will offer some ways through this dilemma later.

The slow crisis

Even more intractable, but less visible than the critical incident, is the 'slow crisis'. This is well-illustrated, if somewhat gruesomely, by the parable of the boiled frog (Box 7.2, taken from Senge, 1990). This phenomenon can concern the group as a whole or, as below, a particular member.

> It continued to be difficult to include Pauline. Generally, she would speak when personally addressed and nodded at other people's comments. She was not generally open to discussing her home life despite agreeing to Paul [co-groupworker] raising some issues during her weekly phone call and visit.
>
> Portfolio P1, 4.1

This 'spectator' phenomenon, in which one or more group members fail to participate or engage to the same degree as the others, is not a dramatic episode but is illustrative of a creeping difficulty which can slowly afflict a group. Without regular reviews by groupworkers, this pattern may remain unrecognised and, therefore, not challenged.

BOX 7.2   PARABLE   OF   THE   BOILED   FROG

Maladaptation to gradually building threats to survival is so pervasive in systems studies of corporate failure that it has given rise to the parable of the 'boiled frog.' If you place a frog in a pot of boiling water, it will immediately try to scramble out. But if you place the frog in room temperature water, and don't scare him, he'll stay put. Now, if the pot sits on a heat source, and if you gradually turn up the temperature, something very interesting happens. As the temperature rises from 70 to 80°F, the frog will do nothing. In fact, he will show every sign of enjoying himself. As the temperature gradually increases, the frog will become groggier and groggier, until he is unable to climb out of the pot. Though there is nothing restraining him, the frog will sit there and boil. Why? Because the frog's internal apparatus for sensing threats to survival is geared to sudden changes in his environment, not to slow, gradual changes.

(From Senge, 1990: 22–3)

RETRIEVAL STRATEGIES

Most groupworkers will try to anticipate, and therefore avoid, difficult situations; however, when they do arise they can provide excellent learning for everyone. In order to achieve this learning, it is important to deploy 'retrieval strategies'. Let us consider what these are and how they can be used to work with the kinds of situations described in the previous section.

Inviting enquiry and dialogue

How can you ensure that you do not have to choose between accommodating, compromising and confronting? What alternatives might there be? Ignoring unacceptable behaviour is to collude with it, but confronting it head on is often to stiffen resistance. Compromising often leads to no-one feeling properly heard. Taking up a position invites opposition and blocks communication. Instead, you should use your authority as a groupworker to invite enquiry and dialogue. You can make your own position clear if this is really necessary, but it should be made plain that this is secondary to the need to explore and enquire. A public statement of anti-racism may ease the conscience, but will serve no useful purpose if it merely confirms and entrenches the racism of the group, now in silent opposition. The group will be experienced as yet another forum where power is used to suppress, even if in these circumstances it is for the right reasons.

As Claire noted in respect of incident #3 (Box 7.1):

> The incident should have been handled in such a way as to avoid a situation of one against the other – I should have drawn Ceiron back to the ground rules of respect, and created an 'us and us', not a 'them and us' situation, using different language. The words I used, 'what you said is offensive', were seen by Ceiron and the rest of the group as provocative.
>
> Portfolio C, 7

Through enquiry you can usually help people to find their own solutions in their own time; in fact, your lines of enquiry will help to speed up this process. Persistent enquiry is a much more challenging experience than a one-line confrontation, with more potential for far-reaching and lasting effects.

Helping the group take responsibility

The dilemma provoked by a critical incident is almost always experienced by everyone in the group as a dilemma for the groupworker. However, it is the group which is experiencing the incident and it should be the group which responds to the dilemma. The groupworker's responsibility is to find ways to help the group accept and act on its responsibilities. This is one of the main purposes of the group, to find ways of supporting one another, if only the workers can avoid putting themselves between the group and its solutions. So, the groupworker's question should not be *what should I do to solve this dilemma?*, but *how can the group find a solution, and how can I best help it to do this?* If the groupworker can don the hat of 'consultant' this helps to make the transition to a different perception of the self in this situation.

The line of enquiry approach begins to involve everyone in the group, rather than provoke a confrontation with one individual. It also involves your co-worker as an enquirer. Rather than the two of you protecting each other in mutual defence, you can each follow the same lines of enquiry with the group in an approach which helps everyone to understand that the workers are exercising their authority *on behalf of the group*. The consequence is that the workers are less likely to feel the kind of inhibition which Jenny felt in incident #6, which led to her avoiding using her authority, to the detriment of both the group and her co-worker. She can use her authority *for* the group not against it.

The elephant doo

Opening up enquiry in the group needs honesty about whatever the difficulty is that the group is experiencing. It will often fall to the groupworker to name this difficulty, because the group is unaware or unwilling to face it. Pointing to the elephant doo in the middle of the group involves some risk, so you should usually reflect on this first with your co-worker where possible, and keep your hypotheses and explanations tentative. You might preface your 'pointing' by commenting on your uncertainty about raising the subject, but that it is a mark of how much trust there is in the group that you feel able to take the risk. If the ground rules anticipated the possibility of pointing at elephant doo, this makes it an easier process because the group will already be familiar with the metaphor and its significance. Even though it is not possible to know exactly what the doo will consist of, how much there will be, when it will arrive and quite what it will smell of, a group that is functioning as more than just a social gathering *will* experience doo. It is really important to anticipate the doo by stating that it will occur and discussing how the group should deal with it when it does.

Pointing at the doo is preferable to leaping into it. In other words, you need to be tentative about any hypotheses you are inclined to make, either about the group as a whole or individual members, as Claire notes:

> Group leaders need to be aware of the need to read between the lines and not always take things at face value … a person not willing to engage in an exercise at the start of the morning session may be because of an argument at home rather due to a 'wilful refusal'.
>
> Portfolio C, 2.1

A note about silence

Silences in groups are often difficult because they can provoke quick judgements about the cause of the silence. Orla records a piece of dialogue in her portfolio which shows her ability to reflect on the silence *with the group*. She speaks out loud what the group members might be feeling, demonstrating the enquiry and dialogue approach, and this leads the group through the difficulty.

Co-worker: So now that we've talked about how we should all act in sessions and what we'll be doing, let's get started.

Orla: First of all, I just want to have a chat as a group to get some ideas of what or who you think a victim is. Any ideas? Don't worry about being too detailed – it's not a test or anything!

Silence.

Co-worker: OK, so what about starting with what might have happened to someone if they are a victim?

Silence.

Orla: Is it that I haven't explained properly, or maybe it's a bit weird having to sit and start shouting things out?
             Sometimes it's tough to think of things under pressure and in front of everyone isn't it?!
             Do you think it might help if Oliver [co-worker] and I started you off with some ideas, then we all write down one idea of our own on a piece of paper, and then read them out together?

Omar: Yes, that sounds alright. It's too weird with everyone staring at you waiting for you to talk.

Portfolio O, 5.2

Where to address the critical incident?

If the group is to learn from an incident or dilemma it needs to be a participant in the aftermath. However, there are times when the immediate response is better made one-to-one with the individual or individuals concerned, rather than in the full glare of the group. This is not an easy decision and you should always check that your decision about where to retrieve the situation is not just a question of where it is *easiest* to do this. We can see Wendy taking herself through all these considerations when responding to Wilma's unassertive and unacceptable aside (Box 7.1, incident #4). Interestingly, Wendy herself uses an aside to deal with the incident:

> On an aside it was explained to Wilma that this comment wasn't acceptable and that during this period of Wanda's life she had been particularly ill. We discussed the fact that everyone has times of their life when their lifestyle or behaviour is not as they would normally wish it to be, and that this is especially the case when someone suffered from a mental illness. Wilma said that she sometimes did things she regretted ... With hindsight, though it may have been appropriate to deal with it in this way at the time, perhaps [I should] have addressed the issue in general terms at the next meeting, referring back to the ground rules ... I wondered if I was copping out by dealing with it outside the group.
>
> Portfolio W, 5.2

Learning from mistakes – time for reflection

I repeatedly (by mistake) called Flo by a different name. Unfortunately it was the name of one of the other group members who has since left and this particular member was held in contempt by the rest of the group due to her brash manner. Flo seemed initially OK about this mistake and reminded me of her name when it happened, however, this became irritating to both of us. It was only when I examined my reasons for the repeated mistake that I was able to rectify this. Flo had the same physical attributes and mannerisms of a neighbour I used to have, the neighbour also had the same name as the other group member, so the two became related.

Portfolio F, 3.3

Names are important and most groupworkers can empathise with Fran's experience above. What is significant for our purposes is the way in which she overcame this mis-association of names. If she had not made the time to reflect on why she was repeatedly making this mistake she may not have become aware of the association of names, and therefore been unable to correct it. Fran's experience illustrates the need for continuing reflection and the importance of learning from mistakes rather than trying to cover them up. It is evident that the experience of writing groupwork portfolios provides this opportunity on a regular basis. (See Malekoff, 1999 and Springer *et al.*, 1999 for further discussion about learning from mistakes.)

BOX 7.3 CHALLENGE WITHOUT ATTACK

Family Support group

When discussing the agenda for future events for the school summer holidays, it was Flo [one of the group members] who suggested it might be good to have days based on different cultures … What emerged from the [Asian theme] session was that the children were very accepting of the day, whereas some of the adults were less accepting, with an attitude of 'I don't know, I don't want to know and I don't care', this being apparent by some of the group's unwillingness to take part in the day's events.

The same attitudes were present at the African Theme Day, with the added comments of 'not this again' … Quite often Flo and Freda would moan loudly about the music being rubbish or the smell of incense being too strong, Freda openly stating that she would not try the food as it 'looked and smelled disgusting'. There were many references to 'Pakis', which I felt could not go unchallenged, and this in turn made people (including me) quite defensive about their position.

Portfolio F, 4.1

ACTIVITY 7.3: NO ACCOMMODATING, COMPROMISING OR CONFRONTING

Consider the situation that Fran describes in Box 7.3, Challenge Without Attack. Write a dialogue which illustrates the way you would like to deal with this situation and which is true to the principles and practices you have learned from reading this chapter; in other words, it opens up lines of enquiry and avoids the 'accommodation–compromise–confrontation' continuum.

KEY POINTS

- There are pitfalls to groupwork practice and it is wise to become aware of those to which you may fall prey.
- Critical incidents and dilemmas in groupwork are actually opportunities for groups (members and workers) to learn more about themselves.
- Too often, the response to a dilemma is to seek to accommodate, compromise or confront – none of these is an adequate response.
- Groupworkers must use their authority to open up a line of enquiry with the group as a better alternative to accommodating, compromising or confronting.
- A key groupwork skill is to help groups take increasing responsibility for working *with* the learning that can arise from a dilemma rather than against it.
- Ground rules should include a section on how the group will work with difficult situations (and 'the elephant doo in the middle of the group' can be an effective metaphor).

FURTHER READING

The following are all articles which focus on issues which are relevant to this chapter. They can all be found in *Groupwork* journal (Whiting and Birch).

Doel, M. (2004) 'Difficult behaviour in groups', *Groupwork*, 14.1, pp. 80–100.
Fatout, M.F. (1998) 'Exploring worker responses to critical incidents', *Groupwork*, 10.3, pp.183–95.
Henchman, D. and Walton, S. (1993) 'Critical incident analysis and its application in groupwork', *Groupwork*, 6.3, pp. 189–98.
Maram, M. and Rice, S. (2002) 'To share or not to share: dilemmas of facilitators who share the problem of group members', *Groupwork*, 13.2, pp. 6–33.
Reid, K. (1988) ' "But I don't want to lead a group!" Some common problems of social workers leading groups', *Groupwork*, 1.2, pp. 124–34.

CHAPTER 8

VALUE

OBJECTIVES

By the end of this chapter you should be able to:

▓ Help individuals in the group to feel valued, and the group to value itself

▓ Enable the group to express its own sense of value and values

▓ Develop explicit and implicit indicators to demonstrate change and movement

▓ Act on information gained about the value of the group

▓ Recognise conflicting values and articulate the group's values when these run counter to the dominant and powerful values.

The many meanings of value are encompassed in this chapter: value, in the sense of appreciating the group and celebrating its successes and a place where people come to value one another; value, as in weighing the costs and benefits of a particular group, evaluating its worth and its impact; and the plural, values, as the source of both potential unity and conflict.

VALUING THE GROUP AND THE INDIVIDUAL

Feeling valued

We noted in Chapter 2 that a group is a place where people can feel that they belong and achieve a sense of meaning. At the heart of this belonging is the feeling of being cared for and valued for who you are. The feeling of being valued seems intangible, but is actually given expression by many small acts, such as having refreshments provided, having others consider your needs and paying respectful attention to what you say, and trusting you enough to challenge you. The sense of feeling valued can have marked effects. One groupworker noted unexpected changes in the group members over the first few sessions, with group members looking smarter and taking more care over their appearance. One of the group members revealed information that was entirely new to the groupworker, even though she had worked individually with this person for more than ten years. Often these feelings are in marked contrast to the experience of not being valued in the wider world.

When group attendance is compulsory, demonstrating that group members are valued is especially important, as Orla notes with the young people obliged to come to the Offending Awareness group:

> I felt that if the young people felt valued and could see the purpose of attending, it would provide more incentive for participation, despite knowing that attendance was compulsory.
>
> Portfolio O, 3.3

In the Parents Plus group, Paul observed a video of one of the group's sessions, and through this window on the group, for the first time he came to realise that the physical environment also reflected a sense of value.

> What struck me most was the display of flipcharts ... consideration needs to be given to producing displays of a better quality – this may assist in conveying to a group how valued they are, where time is taken to produce tools that demonstrate quality. The display in view appears somewhat disorganised.
>
> Portfolio P, 9.1

Group members will attach different value to the opinions of different people. This will depend on the credibility and the perceived power of the person who is doing the valuing. For example, Petra noted the value which one group member, Pat, attached to her sister's opinion.

> Pat got a particular buzz from the shock on her sister's face when she observed her dealing totally differently with the children's behaviour.
>
> Portfolio P1, 5.2

It seems rare for the views of others to be systematically collected, perhaps because it is often practically difficult to do this and also because of ethical and confidentiality issues. More often than not corroborating evidence is likely to be serendipitous. However, there are times when the group members themselves may express a desire to 'take the group to others'. After a particularly exhilarating session, many members of the Offending Awareness group wanted to take copies of the videos which they had made to show members of their family, and even to some of the individuals' social workers (Portfolio O, 4.1). Independent testimony does carry a particular weight, precisely because it is independent. For example, staff in the residential home where Oz was living noted positive changes in his attitude towards staff and residents and his ability to control his anger during minor disputes, and they attributed this to his participation in the Offending Awareness group (Portfolio O, 7.2).

Sometimes the groupworker can experience a dilemma between the value they have for individuals in the group and their concern for the group as a whole. Activity 8.1 will help you consider how you might demonstrate value for both group and individual.

ACTIVITY 8.1: VALUING THE INDIVIDUAL *AND* THE GROUP

Offending Awareness group

> Oz would quite regularly be the first to speak when the group was asked to contribute or begin an activity, which in itself was initially helpful to the group. However, Oz would then continue dominating the conversation, regularly talking over other group members in an effort to be heard and taking centre stage.
>
> Portfolio O, 5.1

Review all the different kinds of activities in Chapter 5 to consider how Orla and her co-worker might demonstrate their value for both Oz and the group.
[Orla's answer to this activity is given in the Appendix.]

In addition to the value which group members derive from the group, they and the group both grow as a result of the value they bring to it.

> It was felt that Oscar had had a positive impact on the group, aside from any impact the group might have had on his personal development.
>
> Portfolio O, 7.2

Difficulties valuing one's self

Group members may find it difficult to value themselves. Lack of confidence and self-esteem may be central to the problems which have led them to become members of the group. This difficulty in valuing oneself can be felt by groupworkers, too, as Jenny reflects in respect of the video of one of the sessions, filmed for inclusion in her portfolio.

> After the initial embarrassment of seeing myself on the video it was difficult to find something positive to say about my performance at first. However, after several viewings I feel that the video extract highlights the cohesiveness of the group and the informal, relaxed setting that has been created.
>
> Portfolio J, 9.1

Small, achievable tasks leading to desired goals will increase levels of self-worth. However, even if there are disappointing outcomes, it is often possible to help the group to value the processes it has experienced and its learning from this.

Celebration

The value of the group can often best be expressed in celebrations. The last session of a time-limited group is especially significant, though the penultimate session can sometimes be more appropriate for an outing, so that the last session returns to the regular pattern of the home base. Planning a celebration is a good opportunity for the group to show its prowess at making a decision, since there are many choices about what form the celebration should take. Paul realised that the co-workers' decision to bring in cakes for the final session of the Parents Plus group, though well-meant, was a missed opportunity for the group to organise this. As it happened, the cakes were 'barely touched' (Portfolio P, 8.1). Samantha's Sound Start group made their decision about how to use the last session in this way:

> The group was asked what they would like to do and they said they wanted to go on an outing together. They wrote a list of the things they wanted to do, such as bowling, ice-skating, cinema and take-away, and then voted for the favourite. This was going to the cinema and then having something to eat.
>
> Portfolio S, 6.2

Every decision calls forth another. Having decided on the cinema, the group had to choose a film, which they did successfully. The group decision-making is also an opportunity for the group as a whole to show its value for individual members.

> The group made sure that the final celebration was a choice which they were all happy with and rejected alternatives on that basis. For example, Stacey did not like swimming because she was afraid of water, so although the others wanted to go they picked something different.
>
> Portfolio S, 6.2

Groups that have no agreed ending, and therefore no last session, need to think how other kinds of event can be celebrated in the group, such as individual birthdays, or even the group's 'birthday'.

INDICATORS

Few would disagree that it is essential to find out whether and how the group is meeting its purposes, but the means and manner of discovery are wide open. Usually the purposes of the group are framed in quite broad terms, so it is useful to help the group think more specifically about what would indicate the group's value.

Individual approaches

An individual evaluation by each group member is a common way to monitor progress session by session. The Parents Plus group used the evaluation format in Box 8.1 (adapted by the co-workers from Webster-Stratton and Herbert, 1994). The co-workers noted that there was evidence that the form was being used with proper discrimination because the questions were rated differently and not ticked off with every question answered 'helpful', which might suggest a stock response. Also, the 'Additional comments' elicited specific information, such as the following:

> 'Useful to be able to spend time discussing issues around last few weeks and topics related to personal situations, rather than sticking to the script.' – *Penny*

> 'I found this session to be a lot better having chatted at the end and calming down made me feel better.' – *Pat*
>
> Portfolio P, 7.1

If the groupworkers take the feedback form seriously, by making sure there is proper time to complete it and by demonstrating that they are acting on the information it contains, the group members are more likely to give considered responses. The group should consider whether it wants individual anonymity, though achieving this can be difficult in a small group or where there are people who need help with reading and writing.

BOX 8.1 FINDING OUT WHAT IS VALUED

Parents Plus group

Parent Programme
Parent Weekly Evaluations

Name _____   Session _____   Date _____

I found the content of the session:

      Not Helpful   Neutral   Helpful   Very Helpful

I feel the video tape examples were:

      Not Helpful   Neutral   Helpful   Very Helpful

I felt the way the group was led was:

      Not Helpful   Neutral   Helpful   Very Helpful

I found the discussion to be:

      Not Helpful   Neutral   Helpful   Very Helpful

Additional comments:

Portfolio P, Appendix

BOX 8.2 FINDING OUT WHAT IS VALUED

Offending Awareness group

Orla received this feedback form from one of the young offenders in the first session of the Victim Awareness block of the Offending Awareness group:

Thinking about the activities you took part in, which of the following did you enjoy most (please circle the number you choose).
① **The Deserving Victim** (game – leader read out newspaper cuttings)
2 **Is it fair?** (matching up statistic cards with sentences)
3 **Hidden victims** (video)
4 **Ice-breaker game** (true/false)
Can you give a reason why you liked it?
Not as boring as sitting around

Circle the activity that you least enjoyed.
1 **The Deserving Victim** (game – leader read out newspaper cuttings)
② **Is it fair?** (matching up statistic cards with sentences)
3 **Hidden victims** (video)
4 **Ice-breaker game** (true/false)
Can you give a reason why this was your least favourite?
Too hard to choose

How well do you think you all worked together as a group? (Circle the number that best describes your feelings.)
1 **Not very well at all**
② **OK**
3 **Really well**
4 **Don't know**
Any reasons for your answer?
Owen was getting on my nerves

If you could change one thing about the session, what would it be?
More games and moving around more

Using the ratings below, how much would you say you enjoyed the session overall?
1 **Not at all**
2 **A little bit**
③ **A lot**

Portfolio O, Appendix

ACTIVITY 8.2: SESSION QUESTIONNAIRES

Offending Awareness group
Consider the information which Orla is seeking from the group members about one of the sessions of the Offending Awareness group (Box 8.2).

- What changes would you make to this questionnaire and why?
- Re-write your revised version.

Group approaches

Probably the most common group approach to evaluating the worth of a session is relatively informal discussion. For example, Jenny noted that everyone in the Memory Joggers group would 'get together as a whole group at the end of each session to discuss the day's events. This has proved especially useful when evaluating feelings' (Portfolio J, 3.2). However, in terms of written formats, the reliance by groupworkers on individual methods to evaluate the group's progress is paradoxical and group methods should be given more consideration, such as participant-focused questionnaires (Adams, 2004). Rather than giving the group a ready-made evaluation sheet, the participant-focused process fully involves the group in the design and application of the questionnaire, including the criteria by which the evaluation will be made. Unlike the pre-prepared questionnaire which is completed as a separate piece to the group session, the participant-focused questionnaire is integral to the group itself. A sense of boredom with the ritual of individual evaluation forms at the end of each session, provoked a creative suggestion for a whole-group approach to evaluation by the Sound Start membership:

> Each session group members completed evaluation sheets. These were anonymous but at the end of the fourth session they said they were bored with them. They asked if it could be done on the flipchart, so I wrote up the sheet and they all completed a big flipchart version in different coloured pens.
> [This was included as an appendix in Samantha's portfolio.]
>
> Portfolio S, 6.1

In the Offending Awareness group, Orla describes a process of valuation which is much more participative and demanding than the 'how was it for you?' approach:

> Group discussion took place at the end of each session. The young people were involved in a 'quick-think' looking back at the initial aims of the session, as recorded on the flipchart, and asked to decide which, if any, activities met which aims and how they did this.
>
> Portfolio O, 7.2

This approach is very leader-led. Group members also need the opportunity to consider what they valued, and did not value, in areas which may not have been related to the aims which were generated by the group leaders.

Indicators and direction

The value of the group can best be demonstrated by an indication of change or *movement*. To know whether there has been movement, we need to know where we started, and to indicate that the movement is desired, we need to know which direction we want to go. These are the specific outcomes (♠ – page 64 in Chapter 4), and they rely on what is often referred to as 'a baseline'. This baseline information should relate to the group's initial purposes and aims, gathered as systematically as possible so that comparisons can be made between the beginning and the end of the group (see Chapter 9).

Endings are often the most visibly unsatisfactory part of the groupwork process, perhaps because the beginnings have been a missed opportunity, or even lost:

> We concluded an exercise on goals towards the conclusion of the first session [of eight] that then got lost. In reviewing our endings, our expectations at the beginning were unavailable.
>
> Portfolio P, 6.2

The Crimestop group systematically asked group members to complete an attitude questionnaire at the beginning and end of their participation in the group, to see whether these changed:

> I don't worry about the consequences of my actions: * SA A N D SD
> I am aware that my offending harms people: SA A N D SD
> If someone ignores me there's no way I can ignore it: SA A N D SD
> It's important to co-operate with others to get what
> you want: SA A N D SD
> Looking after children is a woman's job: SA A N D SD
> etc.
> * SA=strongly agree; A=agree; N=neither agree/disagree; D=disagree; SD=strongly disagree
>
> Portfolio C, Appendix

Attitudinal questionnaires depend on honest and insightful responses and it is problematic to attribute a direct relationship between changes in attitudes and behaviours to the group itself. So, additional methods are needed to weigh the group's impact on a variety of different scales and measures, and produce a more rounded measurement.

If we are to learn how the experience of the group contributed to changes and movement, we need to consider group processes (♦ – page 64 in Chapter 4) as well as specific outcomes. After all, the questions in the Crimestop group questionnaire could have been asked of people who were receiving individual help and none relate to the impact of the group or of groupwork. The measurements of change charted by Helen (below) are less precise, but give us more understanding of the value of the *group* in effecting changes.

> Group members had moved on considerably [by the end of the group]. For example:
>
> 1 Their regular attendance, unless they had a pre-engagement in which case they always phoned or told us.

2 Communication skills improved – they talked with each other and phoned each other outside the group.
3 Group members' mood changed from fear to becoming assertive, making lunch, a cup of tea, deciding which exercise or music they wanted for the relaxation.
4 They were more knowledgeable about their illness and to some degree were able to lessen their [feelings of] guilt by sharing.

Portfolio H, 9.1

Prompted by this question: *If you were to be involved in a similar group soon, what other methods might you use to help group members evaluate the impact of the group on their lives?*, Samantha noted:

I would like to include a method of evaluation which meant the group members could record their initial thoughts on video in the first session and then play them back at the end to see what had changed by the end of the group. I think this would help them to see any changes very clearly and perhaps to see if they have met their own personal aims of being a group member.

Portfolio S, 9.3

Groupworkers should seek creative ways to consider how the group can evaluate itself, making use of group processes themselves.

BOX 8.3 FINDING OUT WHAT HAS BEEN VALUED

Women of Hope group

Evaluation

1 Why did you join this group?
   because I was asked to and also to meet pepole like myself.
2 What were your expectations?
   to try to feel better about my illness.
3 What did you think about the sessions?
   I thought it was interesting.
   a) did it meet your needs? Not all my needs
   b) if not why not? it helped me understand my illness a little better but I feel I didn't get to speak about a lot of things that was a worry to me because there is such a lot of heartache happened in my life and I am only just feeling able to talk about them.
   c) were the sessions long enough? No I feel if they had been longer I could have talked more about things and maybe felt a little better.
   d) the number of sessions? we had eight sessions but I fell we needed about fourteen.

Box 8.3 continued

e) size of the sessions? *I think fourteen sessions would have been better because it would have given the group more chance to say all they needed to.*

4   What did you feel about the group?
I feel that everyone in the group were very understanding and easy to talk to once I got used to them all.

5   What did you like most about the group?
I liked to be able to spend time with people feeling like myself at least now I know I am not by myself.

6   What did you like least?
I liked least the relaxation at the end of the session because I just can't do it no matter how hard I try.

7   What were your expectations?
I learnt that it is better to talk about your problems rather than keep them in as I have done.

8   Give an example where you feel the discussion on depression was helpful to yourself.
I feel it was helpful to me when we talked about death because I don't feel I can talk about what would happen when I die with my family.

9   What did you think of the room e.g.   (a) suitable *but too warm*
                                            (b) unsuitable
                                            (c) alternative

10 Would you join a similar group again?
No because I would have to start from the beginning with strangers which I couldn't do. I was only just getting around to being able to talk about my problems with this group I couldn't start again with strangers.

11 What do you feel should happen now – and why?
I think the group should continue if not at a weekly basis maybe fortnightly if possible.

Portfolio H, Appendix

ACTIVITY 8.3: END OF GROUP QUESTIONNAIRE

Read the completed questionnaire in Box 8.3.

• What information do you think Helen is wishing to gather at the end of the Women of Hope group?
• Judging by the example of a completed questionnaire in Box 8.3, how successfully do you think her questionnaire fulfils its purposes?
• What changes would you make to the questionnaire and why?

Re-write your revised version.
How might revisiting the aims of the Women of Hope group (below, and first presented on page 65) influence the re-drafting of the questionnaire?

♠   We want to be able to go out alone and be confident
♥   We want to feel whole again
♥   We want to feel good about ourselves
♦   We want to share hidden issues
♣   We want to take control of our own lives and gain acceptance.

Explicit and implicit indicators

For a variety of reasons, there are increasing expectations that the notion of value is expressed in very specific outcomes for individuals:

*   Sakhile has moved into her own flat
*   Jane can remember twice as many items on the memory tray
*   Ceiran has not offended again.

Specific outcomes are more easily understood by people who have not taken part in the group itself. Indeed, progress to specific outcomes is very motivating and group members will usually value your help to make their aims more explicit. What does 'feel whole again' (the second aim in the Women of Hope group) mean and how would someone else know that you were feeling whole again? What differences would we see in what you do and say?

Group members will bring concrete examples of changes directly into the group, perhaps adding the testimony of other people outside the group such as family members. These indicators of success are generally well received because the group itself can take some share of the success.

> [In the group] Pat took great pleasure recounting incidents at home when she had acted differently and she got a positive response from her young person. Pat took even more delight when other people such as her sister commented on how differently Pat had behaved.
>
> Portfolio P1, 9.3

At other times it is a fleeting comment which reveals much, all the better when it is a success for the group as a whole. One of the Memory Joggers members exclaims, 'We're getting good!' and laughs out loud at the group's success at a short-term memory game. Another comments that these sessions must be working because the group remembered everything that they had done today.

One problem with relying solely on specific outcomes is their inability to account for the unexpected value which individuals might derive from a group, or the intrinsic value which people experience by *being a group*. Some indicators of success are subtle and could not have been predicted, for example:

> Hayley's behaviour began to change midway, to being a co-operative member of the group. She changed her hair colouring back to its natural colour, her features softened and this was very noticeable to group members who gave her a lot of positive feedback.
>
> Portfolio H, 5.1

'Soften facial features' would be unlikely to have figured in Hayley's list of explicit indicators of success!

One of the indicators which is often used to interpret the success of the group, as opposed to changes to individuals' behaviours, is attendance. This is based on the view that, excluding those who are required to attend, people tend to vote with their feet (Peake and Otway, 1990).

> Josie's attendance is very significant since she has always refused to attend any other groups and often refuses other services. Over the last year she has become a strong member, not in the sense of being dominant but of being stable and being accepted by others … she accepts help from other members.
>
> Portfolio J, 5.1

People's contributions within the group can, in themselves, be a measure of progress.

> Jean feels confident enough to say she has struggled (during the group) and suggest how to improve sessions for her. Jean is now able to make choices for herself.
>
> Portfolio J, 6.2

Many indicators are implicit, and often long term, so that the immediate value of the group is not always evident (Dixon, 2000; Pitts, 1999).

> With groups involving young offenders, one may not always see any positive effects in terms of re-offending until a much later stage in a young person's development.
>
> Portfolio O, 7.2

Group leaders may at first feel puzzled by the ambiguous signals they receive from the group or individual members. Helen and Wendy both noted an ambiguity in the behaviour of a group member:

> Hazel didn't seem to interact with the group. At times she appeared angry and didn't want to be at this group. She didn't sit with the others when they went out for a smoke or chat at interval time. She sat rigid in her chair and would sit in the same position the whole of the time during the session. We noticed she never went for a cup of tea or coffee but would accept it if brought to her. She didn't help with washing up or cleaning anything away … [and yet] Hazel is always ready and makes a special effort with her appearance when I collect her for the group.
>
> Portfolio H, 5.1

> Winsom has consistently remained 'the silent member', although she is the only group member who has promptly attended all sessions.
>
> Portfolio W, 5.1

ACTIVITY 8.4: EXPLICIT AND IMPLICIT INDICATORS

Part one

Consider each of the nine groups which illustrate this book (Boxes 1.C to 1.W).

- Crimestop (Group C)
- Family Support (Group F)
- Women of Hope (Group H)
- Memory Joggers (Group J)
- Managing Behaviour for Carers (Group M)
- Offending Awareness (Group O)
- Parents Plus (Group P)
- Sound Start (Group S)
- Westville Women (Group W)

Explicit indicators are concerned with specific outcomes and, to some extent, contexts (the black suits, ♠ and ♣, as described on pages 64–5). Consider two possible explicit indicators of success for each of the nine groups.

For example, for the Offending Awareness group, one explicit indicator could be a reduction in re-offending and another could be that school attendance rate increases from 50% to a minimum of 70%.

Part two

Consider once again each of the nine groups which illustrate this book.

Implicit indicators are concerned with processes, feelings and other relatively intangible changes (the red suits, ♦ and ♥, as described on pages 64–5, and some contextual factors, ♣, too). Consider two possible implicit indicators of success for each of the nine groups.

For example, for the Offending Awareness group, one implicit indicator could be an increase in communication with family members, and another could be improved ability to make decisions as a group.

Continuation

Evaluations completed during or immediately after a session are sometimes criticised as being 'happy-clappy', completed in the relief which comes from completing a challenging experience. Whatever the value of immediate feedback, it is important to find out what value the group has for people over a period of time.

> Individual [follow-up] interviews enabled us to gain feedback which we hadn't previously known about; for example, one group member told us that she felt stupid doing 'Fruitbowl' [a game], but hadn't felt able to say so at the time.
>
> Portfolio W, 6.P&O

> [At the last session] we all identified a date three months hence when we would meet again as a 'one-off' to review the group from a distance; we booked the venue for the agreed date.
>
> Portfolio P, 6.2

In groups which have a changing membership, or where there are different runs of the group, the workers should consider whether it is appropriate to involve graduates from previous groups to meet the new members. At Oz's last session of the Offending Awareness group, which marked the successful completion of his sentence, he was asked to say a few things about how he felt, and any advice he had for his fellow group members. As part of his personal celebration he was also given the opportunity to choose a follow-up individual activity, in this case a tour of a famous football ground and this gave Orla a chance to catch up with him.

> During our car journey [to the football ground] I asked what he would have changed if he had planned his own ending and how he felt on returning home to his foster carers after the session. Oz provided positive and mature feedback that leaving the group was both positive and memorable, without focusing too much attention on him.
>
> Portfolio O, 6.2

This was just one individual's response, but it helped Orla decide whether this style of ending for individuals in an on-going group should be continued. She gained more information by including an extra question on the group's evaluation sheet about how Oz's leaving had been handled. The members of this group also had the opportunity to discuss their immediate evaluations of group sessions in individual meetings with their caseworkers later. This meant that there was the chance for both an immediate sounding to be taken, and a more considered one, in which the young person was asked to discuss his responses to each question in greater depth, 'thus hopefully uncovering true changes in attitude' (Portfolio O, 7.2).

ACTIVITY 8.5: ACTING ON INFORMATION FROM QUESTIONNAIRES

Offending Awareness group; Women of Hope group
Consider the information which Orla is seeking from the group members about one session of the Offending Awareness group, and that Helen wants about the experience of the Women of Hope group overall (Boxes 8.2 and 8.3).

- What would you do with this information?
- What changes might you make to this or a subsequent group in the light of this information?

In groups which do not have a time limit, regular check-ups are important if the group is not to drift. In the on-going Family Support group, Fran asked all the group members how they saw their own progress as well as the group's. One member's response was:

> I like to support other people and being supported at the same time. I think I have a better outlook on life since attending the group more regularly and look forward to Fridays. It's helped me cope at home a bit better too, I don't get as down when I know that I can talk to someone in the group.
>
> Portfolio F, 9.3

DIFFERENT VALUES

It is likely that there will be different values within the group and frequently a reluctance to face them, or as Fran notes below, a complete denial:

> When we have discussed issues of race in the group, the statement I most frequently hear is 'we don't look on you as being black' which is very difficult to tackle as people do not see this as being a racist statement.
>
> Portfolio F, 8.1

Denying or suppressing differences will not make them disappear, and groupworkers must find ways of helping the group first to recognise and understand them, then to accept them, and if at all possible to enjoy them (see 'Retrieval strategies' in Chapter 7).

Groupwork will quickly expose differences in values between co-workers, too. These may concern 'high order' values, but experience from the Groupwork Project (Box 1.1) suggests that they are more likely to crystallise around 'operational' values. For example, though Samantha and her co-worker, Steve, were at one about the need to strive for anti-oppressive groupwork, they were at considerable odds over the value they each ascribed to the group as a place to have fun, and the group as a forum for learning (the two, of course, are not actually exclusive). Samantha sums up her frustration at the conflict between her desire that the group learn about the topic of the day and Steve's that it should engage in pancake-making:

> Whilst the members had a fun time making pancakes, they were not particularly well-informed about Communication and Continued Learning [the theme of the session].
>
> Portfolio S, 4.1

Other conflicts in value might arise within your team, with others failing to share the value you place on groupwork. Jenny recalls her surprise that some of the health care professionals in her team resented the time being spent on the Memory Joggers group:

> At the planning stage none of us anticipated that we wouldn't receive anything but support and encouragement. I for one didn't anticipate that other professionals would try to hinder, block or belittle our attempts. By not foreseeing this we didn't plan how to handle or answer our critics ... the Clinical Manager claimed the group was affecting our contribution to the

team effort and that the only reason the team is overstretched is that we were spending too much time on our 'tea party'!

Portfolio J, 2.1

Jenny reflects that, with hindsight, she would have had a meeting with all team members (health and social work together) and both managers present in order to discuss the implications of the group and, hopefully, to gain broader support. A planning group could have mobilised this support (see Chapter 3). However, she was able to rectify this later when communicating the effectiveness of the group.

> Colleagues who were initially opposed to the group continuing had a change of heart. They recognised that the group was a worthwhile service and were complimentary in their comments.

Portfolio J, 6.2

Helen, too, was honest about her struggle to advocate for groupwork as a method with other professional groups.

> The group was deemed very low key in the team because I didn't have the time and confidence in a multi-disciplinary setting to be more direct and assertive.

Portfolio H, 2.1

Groups are powerful not just for the group members, but in what groupwork can come to represent in teams and agencies. Differences in working practices are privatised in individual work, unseen and unspoken. In groupwork, however, differences between professional value bases are exposed. An Occupational Therapist approached Jenny because she felt there was a need for an art therapy group for people with dementia, like the members of the Memory Joggers group. An art therapy session was suggested, but the OT said she felt that Memory Joggers was 'not scientific enough' and she would 'run a group of her own which could be clearly evaluated'. This proposed group never materialised.

These differences can be painful at the time. Even so, the discipline of groupwork forces their exposure, with the potential for much more collaborative work in meaningful partnerships.

> Jean's CPN [Community Psychiatric Nurse] says that Jean's attendance has significantly reduced her anxiety levels and has encouraged her to consider other Day Centres, which would help prevent isolation and loneliness ...
> Jane's husband is pleased that she settled in so well and is no longer worried that she is as dependent on him as she once was ...
> John's home carer has telephoned to inform us that John could recall what happened at the session. This is a great step forward for him. Not only has he been able to retain information, his confidence and self-esteem have also increased. John is no longer the shy, nervous person who first attended the group.

Portfolio J, 6.2

Dominant values

> I understand that the Home Office is going to put in place a system of accreditation for Probation groupwork programmes. They will be evaluated as successful if they give value for money and show that by attending, clients' offending rates will reduce ... It could be said that the higher up the hierarchy of management you go in terms of evaluating a programme like Crimestop, money becomes more important and people become less important.
>
> Portfolio C, 6.P&O

Clearly, not only are there different values but these values are held by people with different powers to impose them. The rhetoric suggests that users are at the centre of services, yet the standards and criteria used to judge value are too frequently determined by those who do not experience them in practice. Groupworkers do not have to emulate this; they have the opportunity to move away from rhetoric to provide very real and meaningful exemplars of democratic, participative worlds in which value is not attributed according to hierarchical or budgetary power.

This inclusiveness should be fundamental to the group from its early planning stages. This means reaching out to groups in the community which the agency may be failing to include in its one-to-one or family services. Hand-picked membership tends to perpetuate exclusion. For example, the clientele of the team from whom the Westville Women's group membership was chosen was exclusively white, so the group was white. We know about the low take-up by black people of mental health services. Are there ways in which the group could have reached out beyond the population already served on an individual basis?

Groupworkers have a responsibility to challenge dominant paradigms about what constitutes value in a group, and to help the group to articulate its own versions of value. One valuation almost always begs another; for example, what *is* value for money? A more rounded picture will emerge if valuations are gathered from different sources, such as those suggested in Box 8.4.

BOX 8.4 WHO DOES THE VALUING?

There are many different groups of people and organisations who may have an interest in the group. Which of these 'stakeholders' in the group need to be canvassed to see what value they attribute to the group and its work?

MEMBERS
The people who are regular attenders and feel ownership of the group.

WORKERS
The people who have a role in facilitating or servicing the group.

CARERS
The people who may have responsibilities for the care of group members.

Box 8.4 continued

BACKERS
The people or agencies who have committed time and other resources to the group
– usually colleagues and managers of the workers' agency.

REFERRERS
The people who have suggested that the members might join the group; these people
may continue to work with group members on an individual basis.

HOSTS
The people or organisations who have provided facilities for the group.

OTHERS
Other people with a possible stake in the group, such as other similar groups, the
local community, media, government departments.

KEY POINTS

- A group can enable people to feel valued and to value others.
- Group members are likely to attribute a different 'weight' to the value of other people's opinions.
- Both explicit and implicit indicators should be collected systematically in order to discover what difference the group is making.
- Changes from 'a baseline' tend to be concerned just with individual group members, and the groupworker needs to consider the difference made by the group as a whole.
- Questions about value are not neutral and some are in more powerful positions than others to determine questions such as 'was the group value for money?' Groupworkers must ensure that the group's valuations are articulated as powerfully as possible.

FURTHER READING

These three chapter all appear in a section entitled 'Group work research and evaluation' in Garvin, Gutiérrez and Galinsky (2004). They relate to the North American experience, but have lessons for European and other groupwork. The issues in these chapters also have relevance to the content of Chapter 9.

Brower, A.M., Arndt, R.G. and Ketterhagen, A. (2004) 'Very good solutions really do exist for group work research design problems' in C.D. Garvin, L.M. Gutiérrez and M.J. Galinsky (eds), *Handbook of Social Work with Groups*, pp. 435–46, New York: Guilford Press.
Gant, L.M. (2004) 'Evaluation of group work' in C.D. Garvin, L.M. Gutiérrez and M.J. Galinsky (eds), *Handbook of Social Work with Groups*, pp. 461–75, New York: Guilford Press.
Magen, R. (2004) 'Measurement issues' in C.D. Garvin, L.M. Gutiérrez and M.J. Galinsky (eds), *Handbook of Social Work with Groups*, pp. 447–60, New York: Guilford Press.

CHAPTER 9

GROW

OBJECTIVES

By the end of this chapter you should be able to:

- Evaluate growth in groups and individual members

- Become more self-aware of your own developmental needs as a groupworker

- Understand the significance of the evidence base for groupwork and contribute to it, at least at a local level

- Record groups and groupwork in a systematic way

- Participate in supervision of groupwork

- Contribute to policy development and the establishment of a groupwork service.

GROWING THE GROUP

When we plant a seedling we know the indications for healthy growth. In previous chapters we have considered the conditions for growth – the 'light, water, soil and temperature' of groupwork. In Box 9.1 you will find some key indicators that the group is, indeed, growing. Of course, different groups will have different potential to develop along these lines, so it would be wrong to anticipate that all groups will be able to grow to the same idealised extent. Also, growth is likely to be uneven from session to session. However, *some* growth indicates the group is working, even if this is slow and patchy.

BOX 9.1 SIGNS OF GROWTH: THE GROUP

KEY INDICATORS THAT A GROUP IS GROWING

1 Participation
Group members take part actively in all the group's activities. Discussion is increasingly balanced, so that people who were initially less active in the group become more so.

2 Decision-making
The group is able to develop its decision-making processes so that these are understood and agreed by all the group, and seen as fair. Increasingly, the group refers to these processes to make and review its decisions.

3 Leadership
The group takes increasing responsibility for itself, organising the physical environment, deciding the content, managing itself. Group members are able to make appropriate challenges to the group leadership, and assume authority.

4 Honest communication
Feelings are discussed openly and differences are respected. Members do not avoid conflict, but are able to face it without offence or threat. Taboo issues are opened up, increasingly by group members themselves.

5 Trade
There are increasing levels of 'trade' between the world inside the group and the world outside. That is to say, the growth in the group is reflected in individual members' improved relationships and experiences in their everyday lives.

6 Achievement
Individual members are able to point to specific achievements as a result of their involvement in the group. The group as a whole is able to enjoy these successes and to value the group's contribution to them.

Some of the signs of growth will be apparent at the whole-group level, and others will manifest themselves through the individuals in the group. As an example of the latter, Orla noticed this especially with Omar in the Offending Awareness group; he had been very quiet in the early stages of the group but his participation increased to the extent that he actually volunteered information about a job interview he had recently attended when no-one else in the group responded (Portfolio O, 7.2).

ACTIVITY 9.1: SPOTTING SIGNS OF GROWTH

If you are currently involved in a group, take each of the six indicators in Box 9.1 and apply them to the group. Within each of the six, develop specific indicators which you could use to judge whether and how the group is growing.

If you are not currently involved in a group, complete this same activity by choosing one of the nine illustrative groups as an example (refresh your memory of these groups in Boxes 1.C to 1.W).

Individual and group growth

People come to the group as individuals and they leave as individuals. It is understandable, then, that it is more likely that it is the growth of individual group members which is most evident. The questionnaire which Orla had devised for group members to complete before and after the four sessions on victim awareness frequently provided powerful evidence of individual members' growth over a relatively short period (Box 8.2).

> Staff had expected O'Connor to mess around once video equipment was introduced to the group, but he actually took the exercise seriously and adopted the role of organiser in terms of the sequence of filming and roles allocated ... the feedback noted on his individual case recordings detailed a generally more mature attitude as group sessions progressed.
>
> Portfolio O, 7.2

> Omar's caseworker noted a greater understanding of the implications of offending on the family and society than present at the initial assessment of Omar beginning his involvement with the programme.
>
> Portfolio O, 7.2

The group's growth, as opposed to the individuals', is something which will usually fall to the groupworker to notice and reflect back to the group. Observations like Jenny's below need to be shared with the group itself, since the group might be unaware of how it is changing.

> The group members said they wanted to concentrate some time and energy into being creative and trying out new skills with arts and crafts [in the next session]. This is a far cry from several months ago when decision-making was left to the groupworkers.
>
> Portfolio J, 6.1

Every opportunity should be taken to note the group's growth. It is also worth preparing for the fact that the fruits can sometimes be surprisingly bitter-sweet. Claire's experience of the Crimestop group is not unusual:

> [In the Crimestop group] work done around endings and what they mean takes more than one session and includes some exercises on endings; e.g.

looking at endings as change, as an opportunity rather than as loss. Group leaders have experienced responses akin to those of the bereaved, hostility, withdrawal, lamenting, even suggestions that the group meet up again outside.

Portfolio C, 6.3

Propagating the materials

A very specific opportunity to review and adapt materials arises when a group is repeated with new members. Even when the material is part of an 'off-the-shelf' programme, there are always opportunities for growth by refining and modifying the way the materials are presented. For example, in the Crimestop programme, an exercise asked the group to find words which began with an S, T, O or P to describe their thoughts and feelings, but Claire considered that it would work better without this restriction (Portfolio C, 4.1). Whether the material is home-grown, adapted or off-the-shelf, it needs to be developed in the light of experience. One activity might propagate another, and hybrids will be created as groups make their own changes. Even activities which transplant easily and directly from one group setting to another frequently benefit from some adaptation, such as the Links activity (Box 5.5). Some of the best innovations come from group members' own suggestions, born out of their direct experiences:

> Janice explained that she had found the memory game difficult and made suggestions as to how it could be improved in the future.
>
> *Portfolio J, 8.1*

As we will see in more detail later, it is important to log these experiences carefully so the evidence base for groupwork methods and techniques is systematically collected and reviewed, for groupworkers to benefit from each other's experiences. Unfortunately, when there is pressure on time it is often this systematic recording which is neglected and materials are 'lost'.

> The intended Memory Joggers Information Packs were never completed. I am still undecided as to whether this is important or not.
>
> *Portfolio J, 2.1*

GROWING THE GROUPWORKER

Groupwork is an excellent opportunity for practitioners to develop their own practice. Of course, a group should never be used just as a vehicle for professional improvement; as long as the need for the group has been well researched, the by-product of practice development is justified. Co-workers, in particular, are in a good position to provide feedback to one another, since groupworking provides direct and mutual access to practice. It is better if this feedback is focused, and the key indicators in Box 9.2 should help. They are indications of improvement rather than a set of finishing posts, not absolutes. Groupworkers' opportunities to flourish will vary considerably according to their particular contexts.

BOX 9.2 SIGNS OF GROWTH: THE GROUPWORKER

KEY INDICATORS THAT THE GROUPWORKER IS GROWING

1 Thinking 'group'
   You are able to balance your work with individuals in the group with the group as a whole. You help the group to think of itself as a group, to develop a group identity and group norms. You facilitate the group to take responsibility for itself.

2 Moving to enquiry and dialogue
   You respond to critical incidents in the group with enquiry and dialogue, and are not caught in the accommodation–compromise–confrontation continuum. You are able to enhance the group's insight into its problems and assist its search for solutions.

3 Planning and improvising
   You are prepared to try different methods and techniques in groupwork, make and break patterns, and depart from any 'script' when necessary. You risk moving outside your own comfort zone, which encourages the group to do so, too. You plan well, but can equally abandon these plans when there is a need to improvise.

4 Exercising and relinquishing authority
   You are increasingly able to use your authority on behalf of the group to promote a greater understanding of power, discrimination and oppression in the group and the world outside the group. Equally, you can relinquish authority and find ways which empower the group to exercise authority for itself.

5 Systematic review
   You make time to reflect on the development of your groupwork practice. You learn from mistakes. You read. Your knowledge of groupwork deepens, and knowledge of the evidence-base for groupwork broadens. You write up the group experience in a systematic way for local use and, increasingly, for a wider readership.

6 Thinking groupwork service
   You network with other groupworkers. You take increasing account of contextual factors, making allies of colleagues, managers and the wider community, to develop a higher profile for groupwork. You use the experience of individual groups to promote a groupwork service based on the growing evidence available to you.

Developing your practice requires risk-taking and acknowledgement of the growing pains which accompany this. Groups that are doing 'just fine' and groupworkers who experience no challenge or frisson from their groupwork are likely to have become stuck without being aware of the fact (see Box 7.2).

Self-awareness

Groupworkers need to use a systematic framework to capture their groupwork and to reflect on it, such as a groupwork portfolio (see Chapter 1). The process of compiling a portfolio as part of a programme for continuing professional development helped the practitioners in the Groupwork Project (Box 1.1) to reflect on their own growth as groupworkers, and supported them to venture out of their comfort zones (Doel *et al.*, 2002). This relates particularly to the fifth key indicator, systematic review (Box 9.2). Groupworkers in the project reported the positive effect of specific questions which acted as signposts through the portfolio. Examples are:

> *5.1 Individuals in the group (§3 Reflection)*
> [Following your description of some examples of different kinds of behaviour in the group] how did the individuals' behaviour make you feel? If you could script your response how would it differ from the reality of what happened?
> *7.2 Evaluation (§3 Reflection)*
> In what ways has the group worked *as a group,* as opposed to a collection of individuals? What part do you feel you have played in helping the group achieve its purposes?
> *8.1 Anti-oppressive groupwork (§3 Reflection)*
> In what ways was your own biography similar or different to group members' and what was the impact of these similarities and differences?
> *9.1 Video (§2 Analysis)*
> How does what you see yourself doing in the video extract [of the group session] relate to your understanding of groupwork theory and practice?
> *9.3 The group members speak (§3 Reflection)*
> If you were to be involved in a similar group soon, what other methods might you use to help group members evaluate the impact of the group on their lives?
> from Doel and Sawdon's *Groupwork Portfolio* (Doel *et al.*, 2002)

The signposted portfolio helps to steer practitioners away from bland general statements towards more specific detail. For example, a statement of general self-affirmation, such as 'I feel that this was done in a very anti-oppressive manner' becomes 'I showed inclusive behaviour by getting everyone to sit around the table and by explaining the exercise to Sian so that she had no reason not to join in' (Portfolio S, 8.1). Trigger questions in the portfolio are designed to help groupworkers become more critical and to make statements which it is possible to verify or falsify.

Let us consider the growth of some of the groupworkers you have come to know during the course of the book. Fran notes the following about herself:

I am aware that I am exactly the same in the group as I am with individual service users – that is, I find it difficult to draw to a close. I am working on my summarizing skills in order to draw to a successful conclusion.

Portfolio F, 5.2

Claire develops a better understanding of the meaning of the group's resistance:

I have learned to view resistance from the group and group members as an integral part of the group life and not personal to me.

Portfolio C, 2.1

Paul reflects on how a difficult session ending provoked better ones in the future:

The rushed end to session three led to a deliberate focus on managing conclusions more effectively, an experience of active learning.

Portfolio P, 5.2

Orla notices an improvement from the first to the second run of the Offending Awareness group:

I became more adept at tuning in and recognizing anxiety, frustration, uncertainty.

Portfolio O, 3.2

Groupworkers whose practice is developing well will also become aware of the missed opportunities and rehearse ways in which similar opportunities will not be missed in future. Jenny comments on such an occasion:

Josie is no longer a silent member and has openly stated that the 'people in our group are nice'. This was a missed opportunity on our part. Rather than bringing this into the forefront, we gushed and let the moment pass. It would have been interesting to hear how other members viewed the group.

Portfolio J, 2.1

It is also illuminating to consider what signs there might be that growth is not occurring. For example, novice groupworkers are prone to behave as if they are another group member, and we would expect to see this changing over time. The groupworker in Activity 9.2 (not one of those from the illustrative groups) 'rescues' one of the group members by deploying the same unhelpful behaviour as the person from whom he considers she needs rescue. The group in question is, in fact, a team of workers.

ACTIVITY 9.2: SPOTTING LACK OF GROWTH

Gillian stated 'I have contacted his social worker, Sharon James'. She had stated the wrong person as social worker and was quickly corrected about the right name of the social worker. The group member who interrupted her then carried on the conversation. As the group leader I interrupted the group member who had interrupted Gillian and allowed Gillian to carry on with her conversation.

Portfolio X, 5.2

• Why is this not a helpful intervention by the groupworker?
• How might the groupworker have intervened more skilfully? (Think especially of key indicators of growth #1 and #2 in Box 9.2.)

GROWING THE EVIDENCE BASE

We do not have sufficient empirical research on group work to support a strong foundation for evidence-based practice.

(Garvin *et al.*, 2004: 6)

Garvin *et al.*'s (2004) comments are apt, but by no means confined to groupwork and they focus on just one facet of knowledge, empirical research (see Chapter 2). Systematic reviews of the effectiveness of groupwork are relatively rare but encouraging; for example, Barlow's (1997) study found that group-based programmes produced better results than individual programmes in improving children's behaviour problems. There is no doubt, then, that the search for the 'knowledge crystals' (Preston-Shoot, 2004: 19) is critical so that we can know more about what works, the gaps in our knowledge, and gain better understandings of the experience of groupwork (Tolman and Molidor, 1994). This will strengthen the theoretical foundations of groupwork and build accountable and ethical practice, all leading to improvements in practice (Gant, 2004; McDermott, 2005; Pollio, 2002). This is important if we are to develop standards for groupwork and influence policy makers to promote groupwork as a mainstream service (AASWG, 1999).

Whose evidence?

What counts as evidence and who does the counting is a highly contested area, as we saw in Chapter 2. For example, in the field of youth justice, Yates (2004) asks us to beware of single, stark measures of success such as re-offending rates, and reminds us of existing evidence, too often conveniently overlooked, about deprivation and disadvantage. True to the principles advanced throughout this book, the group itself should be the principal deciders of what counts as evidence. Helping the group to articulate this is one of the groupworker's key tasks, but how might this best be done?

Fortunately, groupworkers in general and social workers in particular have skills and experience which mirror qualitative research methods – attending to process and meaning, observation and interviewing, etc. Indeed, the context of much research is in groups, such as the focus group. Seen in this light, the groupworker is an 'insider' researcher-practitioner and each group is, or has the potential to be, an example of research-in-action (McDermott, 2005). Moreover, 'outsider' researchers are likely to focus only on individual outcomes from a group, whereas insiders appreciate the significance of using *the group* as a unit of research. 'Studies conducted by uninvolved researchers are much more likely to present data on individual members, than on the group as a whole' (Johnson *et al.*, 2001: 68).

In the language of research, each group is a single case design. The opportunity to exploit this potential is often missed, so Johnson *et al.*'s (2001) account is welcome as a practical framework for groupworkers. For example, in one account, group members were presented with material about their own group in graph form, such as attendance patterns and the increase in the number of individuals who speak from session to session. The group's response was very positive, since it graphically increased their understanding of themselves as a group. Researcher and groupworker are one and the same person, so that 'it didn't feel as if I was doing research' (*ibid.*: 68). Groupworkers can use their expertise and experience to help group members develop a base-line of information at the beginning of the group or even prior to this, so that comparisons can be made during and after the group. Of course, measuring is a culturally specific practice and it is important that these base-lines are determined by group members. For example, few western groupworkers would expect to hear the main problem as 'feeling far from God' (and, therefore, unlikely to construct the baseline question, 'how far or near do you feel from God?); yet this is what a Botswanan woman described when asked what her physical symptoms were.[1]

A local evidence base

Findings by Preston-Shoot (2004) echo those of a decade earlier by Forte (1994), in which the majority of journal articles on groupwork 'were not research based but were descriptions of practice ... suggesting little contribution to the knowledge base of social group work' (Mayadas *et al.*, 2004: 49–50). However, single accounts of groupwork have much to offer and, realistically, are all that practitioners have the resource to gather. Practitioners rightly expect support in order to make the push from doing everyday practice to gathering information in a systematic fashion to develop the evidence base. Fran's experience is, sadly, not unusual:

> The recording of the sessions was only decided once I had enrolled on the groupwork course, and prior to this no recording took place.
>
> Portfolio F, 7.1

Practitioners' accounts *do* need to be more systematic if they are to serve a wider purpose, as outlined in Chapter 1. Fortunately, methods of groupwork evaluation have strong parallels with qualitative research methodology, and these should help broaden the groupworker's approach to data collection and avoid defensive evaluations, in which the pressure to prove good outcomes overcomes a genuine spirit of enquiry (O'Connor, 1992). Evaluation training can help groupworkers become aware of the proper limitations of the conclusions they can draw, as Orla notes in these two portfolio entries:

> Methods of evaluation cannot always provide specific insight into whether progress has been a direct result of groupwork alone or should be evaluated within the wider context.
>
> Portfolio O, 7.2

Unfortunately, Omar re-offended and is no longer with our team, thus making evaluation of further change difficult. However, Omar's mother did believe that generally Omar had seemed more communicative at home since working with the team.

Portfolio O, 7.2

Omar's mother (above) provides one element in the 'triangulation' of evidence, in which groupworkers seek to gather data from a variety of sources (see Box 8.4). Moreover, we can see how Orla's understanding that evaluation does not end with the group is tempered by the everyday difficulties which practitioners face in tracking service users.

What is it realistic to expect groupworkers to contribute to the evidence base? In Box 9.3, I indicate how a *local* evidence base might be a practical way forward, not out of parochialism, but as a realistic prospect, with the added value that it is likely to be in tune with the local context. The experience of portfolios as a systematic, standardised and confidential means of collecting and presenting evidence is a sound foundation for such a local evidence base (Doel *et al.*, 2002).

Progress in group work or, for that matter, in any form of professional practice is rooted both in the wisdom of its practitioners as they reflect on their professional actions and in the careful collection of data about the impact of the practice on members and their environments.

(Garvin *et al.*, 2004: 3)

BOX 9.3 SIGNS OF GROWTH: THE LOCAL EVIDENCE BASE

KEY INDICATORS THAT THE LOCAL EVIDENCE BASE IS GROWING

1   Groupworker-researcher
    Groupworkers begin to see themselves as 'insider' researchers and note the parallels between group and research processes; each group is seen as a 'single-case design'.

2   Baselines
    Groupworkers systematically gather baseline information early in the group, so that comparisons can be made later, and also after the group. Groupworkers triangulate their evidence; that is, they take evidence from a number of sources over a period of time (group members, family members, other professionals, etc).

3   Broadening range of evaluation models
    Groupworkers do not confine themselves to empirical methods, but use a range of models, including empowerment models to enable the group itself to articulate what counts as meaningful evidence.

Box 9.3 continued

4   A local database
    Information about each group is systematically presented, so that there can be meaningful learning across groups. The (anonymised) information is available to others – groupworkers, other practitioners, users of the agency's services, managers – perhaps via a website or web pages on the agency's site.

5   Theorising from practice
    Groupworkers begin to see themselves as practical theorists, articulating the theoretical basis for their practice and using their groupwork experience to develop theory.

6   Publication
    Some accounts of groupwork, systematically evaluated, are written for formal publication by groupworkers, group members or a combination. Local evidence bases link up to develop wider networks.

Links between local evidence bases and with the formal literature would build a strong network of practice knowledge, a 'community of practice' (Wenger *et al.*, 2002) with appropriate links to a national body such as the Social Care Institute for Excellence (SCIE). The 'bottom-up' nature of its growth would be more likely to give this evidence base the credibility and accessibility which is so important if evidence is to be translated into daily practices. We would hope to see not just groupworkers, but group members encouraged to publish their own accounts, something which remains very rare (The Thursday Girls, 2004).

GROWING THE GROUPWORK SERVICE

If groups and groupwork can make a difference to the people who experience them, it follows that we should find ways to help agencies to develop groupwork as an integrated and regular feature of its services. There are four pillars necessary to support this:

*   systematic recording
*   groupwork education
*   supervision of groupwork
*   policy development.

Systematic recording

If groupwork is making a difference, we need reliable and detailed information about this 'difference' in order to build a case for a sustained groupwork service. This information must be gathered and presented systematically, starting with the detail of each group session. Memories can be unreliable, so it is important to take soundings as soon after the experience of a group session as possible. The diagrammatic format of a group 'snapshot' (Boxes 9.4 and 9.5) was developed in the Groupwork Project (Box 1.1) and was successful in helping patterns to be recognised and changes to be noted. These build into an album of the group's progress. In addition, changes in individual members' attitudes, behaviours and circumstances need to be documented and presented in a confidential manner (Northen, 2004). The groupworker's recorded commentary on the specific difference that groupwork has made is the final layer in this process.

The group should be central to decisions about what use will be made of information about the group as a whole and about its individual membership. This means an open consideration of the means by which the knowledge that is derived from the group is to be put to best use (for example, in groupworkers' portfolios and policy documents for the agency), whilst respecting privacy. How we record the group is a measure of how it is valued and methods must be participative and empowering.

ACTIVITY 9.3: SELF-PORTRAIT

Westville Women's group

> I think it would have been a good idea to set aside time at the end of each session for the whole group to fill in the snapshot [Box 9.4]. Individuals would have become more aware of both their own and other contributions and it would have given a more immediate response to the 'feel' of the session.
>
> Portfolio W, 6.1

Rather than a private event between co-workers after a session, how might the taking of the group snapshot become a group activity, thus putting Wendy's good intention into actual practice?

Finding accessible ways of recording in which all group members can feel they have a stake might require other media, such as audio-vision or a group diary. It will mean respecting the group's decisions about the uses to which information about the group will be put, though Samantha's experience was a common one, with members genuinely supportive about sharing the group's experience for educative purposes, as long as confidentiality was assured. Samantha ensured that all of the recording for the Sound Start group was completed during the sessions themselves – on flipcharts, evaluation sheets, handouts, homework sheets and the Group Agreement (Portfolio S, 7.1).

> I mentioned that I am doing a groupwork training course, so I would be writing about the group and videoing a session. I asked whether they [the group members] were OK with this and they all said that they were.
>
> Portfolio S, 3.3

Any products from the group are also a record of work. For example, the Offending Awareness group constructed a flipchart picture of a person and drew on this outline the different ways in which anger might be experienced: a lump in the throat, churning

BOX 9.4 GROUP SNAPSHOT

Name of the group: My name:
Session number: Date:

| GROUP PICTURE
Who was present and who sat where: | Was anyone absent?

Is there a need to follow up?

Who contributed most – least?

Is there a pattern? Where does power lie in the group? |

| AIMS
The main aims of the sessions were:

1

2

3 | THEMES
The themes that are emerging are: |

What was the general atmosphere and feeling of this session of the group?

What was my main contribution and what did my co-leader contribute?

What I learned most from this session as a groupworker was ......

Future plans include ......

BOX 9.5 GROUP SNAPSHOT

Name of the group: Sound Start
Session number: 1

My name: Samantha
Date: 21 February

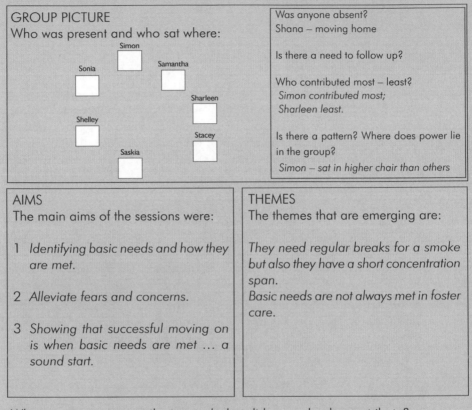

GROUP PICTURE
Who was present and who sat where:

Simon
Sonia
Samantha
Sharleen
Shelley
Stacey
Saskia

Was anyone absent?
Shana – moving home

Is there a need to follow up?

Who contributed most – least?
Simon contributed most;
Sharleen least.

Is there a pattern? Where does power lie in the group?
Simon – sat in higher chair than others

AIMS
The main aims of the sessions were:

1 *Identifying basic needs and how they are met.*

2 *Alleviate fears and concerns.*

3 *Showing that successful moving on is when basic needs are met ... a sound start.*

THEMES
The themes that are emerging are:

They need regular breaks for a smoke but also they have a short concentration span.
Basic needs are not always met in foster care.

What was my main contribution and what did my co-leader contribute?
The Jenga game – trying to explain a fundamental concept to the group making it understandable and fun, also managing constant interruptions and diversions.
Sonia [co-worker] was good at managing interruptions while she was explaining the Storyboard exercise. She put it to them in a way they could grasp and in the context of what they are learning.

What I learned most from this session as a groupworker was ......
Some interruption is good because it shows they are listening and want to be involved – and that they 'own' the group. There comes a point when it is too much and the point of the exercise is lost. This didn't happen, but it could do.

Future plans include ......
To be aware of Simon's power in the group and to make sure he sits on a lower chair, preferably sofa. To play more music as requested in evaluation sheets.

stomach, clenched fist, etc. This is a graphic record of the group's discussion. This same group used a camcorder, again a form of record of the group's activity (which several members wanted to show their families and social workers). Orla designed a form which each group member completed both at the beginning and at the end of the particular sequence on victim awareness, to see whether there were any changes in attitudes as a result of the group sessions.

However, some practitioners' room for manoeuvre is curtailed when it comes to recording the group and its work:

> There was not a lot of choice open to us as to how we decided to record our
> groupwork. It is laid down in Probation Service policy.
>
> Portfolio C, 6.1

Groupwork education

Sustaining groupwork practice and learning requires a commitment to continuing professional development. In the Groupwork Project (Box 1.1), training and education in groupwork was available to practitioners pre- and post-qualification and some students on placements were also involved in the groups. National occupational standards in England and Wales ensure that groupwork is a requirement of qualifying training in social work (TOPSS, 2002) and it is crucial to ensure that the next generation of social workers are groupwork literate (Birnbaum and Wayne, 2000). The training arm of the Groupwork Project was evidently a significant factor in initiating and sustaining the groups (Doel and Sawdon, 1995), as Helen remarked:

> The Group Skills training programme was the deciding factor to enable me
> to pursue the group at this time.
>
> Portfolio H, 2.1

Having an assessed component to a groupwork module as part of a larger programme of continuing professional development helps to anchor the place of groupwork alongside required statutory training. Of course, practitioners who do not have access to these kinds of opportunity must consider how to create peer support, perhaps lobbying for groupwork education to be made available. Helping agencies to understand the connection between groupwork and better teamwork is one way forward. A regular forum to share group experiences and critical incidents can be a strong support (Gould and Masters, 2004).

Writing about practice helps to understand it (Walker, 1985), and portfolios can accelerate this understanding, depending on how they are structured. The 'knock-on' effect of having to work on a portfolio can be seen in Jenny's confession:

> Once our portfolios were completed, we [the group leadership of four] ceased
> to meet up at the end of sessions to discuss the day's events. I didn't appreciate
> how important this stage was, or how relevant to the group's development,
> until this happened.
>
> Portfolio J, 7.1

Many of the groups in the Groupwork Project (Box 1.1) brought staff together who were at different stages of professional education, with considerable benefits in terms of informal coaching and mentoring. The impact on the support workers in the Memory Joggers group was notable:

> Our support workers, Julie and Joy, have renewed confidence in their abilities and are both now taking part in an Open University course.
>
> Portfolio J, 6.2

Training and education frequently uses a group as a context for learning, even if groupwork is not the content or focus, since 'explicit and implicit learning are likely to occur through participation in group activities' (Eraut, 2005: 1). The omnipresent use of small and large groups in continuing professional development strengthens the case that becoming 'group literate' is likely to benefit all training events.

Supervision of groupwork

A groupworker's supervisor does not necessarily have to be an expert in groupwork, but they should be able to coach, mentor and facilitate (Parsloe and Wray, 2000). Supervisors can keep pace with a group's progress via recording, which can help supervisors prepare for supervision sessions. Feedback on portfolio work, along with consultation from experienced groupworkers, can promote new options, even when these might seem obvious:

> Until we had the second groupwork consultation, we [co-workers] hadn't considered a formal ending to our sessions. It was recommended that we all finish the session together; initially we hadn't and there had been a sense of unfinished business when members drifted away separately. Members arrived separately, but we always made a point of beginning the group together. Finishing together warrants the same consideration.
>
> Portfolio J, 6.1

Supervisors in touch with groupwork are more likely to be committed to helping it become part of a mainstream service (Doel and Sawdon, 1995) and a manager's support can be critical, as both Orla and Jenny describe:

> From the outset, the manager had identified the possibility of beginning groupwork within the team and proposed that members of the team holding case responsibility for young people should take on the role of researching and implementing the overall [group] programme.
>
> Portfolio O, 2.1

> [My manager] feels that because the group has been successful and is well established the opportunity is there for Outreach [another service to people with dementia] to continue with Memory Joggers, allowing it to run

permanently. In the next few weeks we will have to open this idea to group members and gradually introduce workers from Outreach.

Portfolio J, 6.2

One of the greatest services a supervisor can provide is to take sufficient interest in a supervisee's practice to observe it and comment (Wayne and Cohen, 2001; Le Riche and Tanner, 1998). Social work students will have experience of live observation in their qualifying training, and candidates compiling a portfolio are often *obliged* to seek this, but it is good practice to establish regular observation, required or not, with proper permissions from group members. Comments from some of the supervisors' reports in the Groupwork Project portfolios are collected in Box 9.6. Co-workers need to decide whether it will be better to have the same or different supervisors, if this choice is available to them.

BOX 9.6 GROUPWORKERS OBSERVED

Women of Hope group

Before the group moved on to new issues Helen summarised the previous input, highlighting the common themes of the group and drawing individuals together through common ground.

report in Portfolio H, 9.2

Flipchart papers from past sessions were posted around the room displaying the group's earlier sessions. Helen used these to highlight areas covered in previous weeks.

report in Portfolio H, 9.2

I found observing this group session a positive experience. The group had obviously developed in such a way that a safe environment was able to facilitate individual growth. All group members felt the group had been a good, although sometimes challenging, experience.

report in Portfolio H, 9.2

Parents Plus group

Paul connects previous experiences of the group with the present discussion … He comments on a difference a group member discloses about her behaviour, with Paul linking this back to a learned skill … Paul brought in another group member to comment on an account given that was self-blaming to encourage a challenge to this negative story.

report in Portfolio P, 9.2

I felt privileged to see two skilled workers.

report in Portfolio P, 9.2

Policy development

To establish and sustain a successful groupwork service, an agency must pursue policies to promote it. Mechanisms are needed to feed the experiences of individual groups to policy makers in the agency. Agencies vary widely in the effectiveness of their information systems and most are some distance from establishing accessible databases to provide the kind of local evidence base described earlier in this chapter. Frontline groupworkers might understandably feel that they cannot concern themselves too deeply with system-wide matters, though they can ensure that their immediate colleagues are within the group's 'footprint', and that reliable information is available to those senior managers who will carry a torch for groupwork.

These champions need documentation about which purposes groups can meet that cannot be met in other ways, or that are better met through groupwork. The group snapshots, taken together with a portfolio of groupwork practice where this is available, can be used as the basis for an executive summary for busy senior managers. A sample of portfolios might also be made available to agency policy makers to keep them in touch with the impact of practice on the agency's users. The group members might write a letter or perform a presentation. Certificate ceremonies are another way of highlighting and rewarding good practice with groups. Agency champions may not completely arrest the following kinds of comment, but they can help to check them:

> Colleagues attending the Skills in Groupwork course heard their participation
> in groupwork described as 'a luxury'.
>
> Portfolio P, 2.1

As well as information flowing up and down the agency, it is important that experiences of groupwork travel *across* the agency to encourage educational transfer, in which practitioners can access each other's learning:

> As a result of Memory Joggers, support workers from other teams have
> expressed a desire to run a similar group in their area.
>
> Portfolio J, 6.2

Agencies may need to be alerted to an understanding of how groupwork can help meet their main concerns. The link between groupwork skill and good teamwork, and the directives from government for inter-professional working to break down barriers between agencies are just two examples. Workers with different professional backgrounds can co-work a group as part of this kind of initiative, as Helen and the Community Psychiatric Nurse demonstrated with the Women of Hope group (Box 1.H). Inter-professional support was evident at a basic resource level in the Memory Joggers group, with the donation of regular refreshments by the Health Service Clinical Manager (Portfolio J, 2.1), in a situation which moved from open hostility to one of active support for the group. There are many ways in which an agency can be alerted to the wider value of a groupwork service (see Activity 9.4).

ACTIVITY 9.4: GROUPWORK CHAMPIONS

Which of these factors is likely to attract champions for groupwork at a senior level in your agency? Give each one a score out of 5 (0 = not at all persuasive, to 5 = highly persuasive) and add any other factors about groupwork which you think might be attractive to the agency's senior management team.

- Groupwork can provide a service to more people at one time than individualised forms of work
- Groupwork can enhance the quality of the agency's services, empowering service users by meeting other people in similar circumstances
- Groupwork is more transparent than individual work
- Groupwork can support mentoring and coaching, with more experienced staff helping to develop less experienced colleagues as co-workers
- Groupwork skills and experience ('group literacy') benefit teams and teamwork, and are likely to help staff morale
- 'Group literacy' is necessary to make best use of all forms of continuing professional development and other forms of staff development
- Groupwork could be used to supervise staff, with group supervision supplementing individualised forms of supervision
- Groups can provide aggregated information about large numbers of service users
- Evaluation methods in groupwork are often more transparent, robust and systematic than individualised evaluations
- Groups can be co-led by staff from different agencies and different professional backgrounds, thus encouraging inter-professional and inter-agency working.

Agency backing often makes the difference. Paul's experience of co-working the Parents Plus group was notably different from his previous experiences of 'one-off' groups:

> What I have learned from being a part of a wider, officially sanctioned initiative is that it feels supportive, and this instils confidence.
>
> Portfolio P, 2.1

All of the elements we have explored in this chapter will help to amplify the benefits from one single group. The possibility of a groupwork service brings these benefits to many more people. Without losing the attraction of the 'difference' which groupworkers and members experience, we need to bring it into the mainstream so that so many more people can experience its power and creativity.

KEY POINTS

- Indicators help to assess whether and how the group, the group members and the group worker are growing.

- Groupworkers have skills that are similar to those of researchers, which puts them in a good position to develop the evidence base for groupwork.
- Networking in order to grow a local evidence base is a good place to start, and this requires systematic recording of groups and groupwork.
- 'Group literacy' helps many aspects of an agency's work, including teamwork and all aspects of continuing professional development; however, most agencies need to be alerted to the broader benefits of groupwork.
- It is important to grow from *ad hoc* groups to a groupwork service, whilst maintaining the creativity of groupwork at the service level.

FURTHER READING

All of these journal articles take the themes raised in this chapter further.

Brower, A.M., Arndt, R.G. and Ketterhagen, A. (2004) 'Very good solutions really do exist for group work research design problems' in C.D. Garvin, L.M. Gutiérrez and M.J. Galinsky (eds), *Handbook of Social Work with Groups*, pp. 435–46, New York: Guilford Press.

Johnson, P., Beckerman, A. and Auerbach, C. (2001) 'Researching our own practice: single system design for groupwork', *Groupwork*, 13.1, pp. 57–72, Whiting and Birch.

McDermott, F. (2005) 'Researching groupwork: outsider and insider perspectives', *Groupwork*, 15.1, pp. 91–109, Whiting and Birch.

Pollio, D. (2002), 'The evidence-based group worker', *Social Work with Groups*, 25.4, pp. 57–70, Haworth Press.

Preston-Shoot, M. (2004) 'Evidence – the final frontier? Star Trek, groupwork and the mission of change', *Groupwork*, 14.3, pp. 18–43, Whiting and Birch.

FOOTNOTE

1 From a portfolio in England for the Advanced Award in Social Work (AASW).

EXAMPLES OF RESPONSES TO ACTIVITIES

ACTIVITY 3.1: THE PLANNING GROUP

1 Which key people should be members of the planning group for your proposed group (in addition to yourself)?

- Manager (and/or supervisor/senior practitioner) to 'clear a way' within the agency to make sure the group has the backing of the agency and is adequately resourced.
- A 'consultant' – perhaps a practitioner who has experience of running similar groups.
- A colleague from the team who may help to spread support for the group within the team and help with the logistics.
- Possible colleagues from other agencies (domestic violence unit, etc) who can provide advice or possible help with recruitment.
- Service users (see question 3 below).

Need to make sure that the planning group is a manageable size and is focused on this particular group. A larger group might be appropriate to develop inter-agency groupwork (a planning committee), but the specific planning group needs to be a workable size – perhaps four to six?

2 What tasks would the planning group have?
- Logistics, such as finding and deciding a venue, transportation, budget, etc.
- Recruitment and publicity; deciding best methods to recruit members to the group.
- Shape the overall remit of the group – its purpose, aims and objectives (though these are likely to be re-shaped by the group itself).
- Helping to plan some of the content of the group sessions.

- Be involved in the evaluation process, ensuring that evaluation takes place from the start of the group.
- Involvement in dissemination of the group's experience (safeguarding confidentiality).

3   How will potential group members be included in the planning group?
- A service user 'consultant' – perhaps a service user who has successfully been through similar kinds of experience (or a group like the one proposed).
- A 'representative' of the kind of people likely to be recruited to the group.
- Evaluations from previous groups of this kind.
- A survey of potential group members to find out what they would like.

ACTIVITY 5.5: FIT FOR PURPOSE

It is important to consider each activity carefully. How does it meet this group's particular purposes at this particular time? Check, for example, that an ice-breaker hasn't become just habitual or a personal favourite of one of the group leaders! Consider the ice-breakers, warm-ups and cool-downs in Box 5.6, and the activities in Box 5.7.

Which kinds of purpose might each of these different activities fulfil for the group? From this, you should develop criteria which you could use to help you consider what kind of activity to introduce into the group and when.

Getting to know each other	Encouraging self-disclosure	Having fun
Setting the tone	Breaking down barriers	Leading into the group's work
Modelling behaviour	Shaking the group up	Focusing (e.g. on a particular skill)
Building confidence	Building group identity	Sharing power
Energising	Getting physically close	Creating balance
Relaxing	Bringing in potential silent members	Reconnecting with each other
Releasing anxiety		
Removing inhibitions		
Expressing feelings		

[Responses from a workshop in the Groupwork Project (Box 1.1).]

ACTIVITY 6.2: THE POWER OF REWARD

Sound Start group

I was very proud of Sharleen, given her learning difficulties and how difficult she had found it to attend the first session, and this was 'named' outside the group setting and sometimes during the session. When Sharleen was working

Activity 6.2 continued

hard I would name it by saying something like, "Sharleen seems to be doing a good job on her handout. That's really good."

Portfolio S, 5.1

What are the benefits of rewarding Sharleen in this way?

Sharleen's confidence increases. This might help her to contribute more in the wider group. She will see the group in a positive light and feel that it is a good place to be.

What are potential risks of this?

Other group members might feel envious of this attention or feel excluded. This might make them feel and act negatively towards Sharleen.
Other group members might see the group leadership as partisan.

How might this reward be complemented with a reward for the group as a whole?

Remarking on the supportive atmosphere of the group which has enabled Sharleen to do so well.
Asking others in the group how they feel Sharleen is doing (this has some risks).

ACTIVITY 8.1: VALUING THE INDIVIDUAL *AND* THE GROUP

Offending Awareness group
How might Orla and her co-worker demonstrate their value for both Oz and the group in this situation:

Oz would quite regularly be the first to speak when the group was asked to contribute or begin an activity, which in itself was initially helpful to the group. However, Oz would then continue dominating conversation, regularly talking over other group members in an effort to be heard and taking centre stage.

Portfolio O, 5.1

Orla's Answer to Activity 8.1

Oz had spent the past four years of his life living in a residential home for young people displaying challenging behaviour, with between three and six other residents, and so was used to being in a group environment with peers. It became clear that he had learned that one must make one's mark in such group situations or else someone else may dominate, making life difficult. Oz's experience of peer interaction involved the need to speak very loudly and take control of a situation from the start to ensure a respected place in the group.

Knowing that Oz responds well if treated fairly and addressed in a non-confrontational manner, we agreed that the best way to deal with this would be to gently address the behaviour, for example by thanking him for his contribution, followed by asking a different group member for their thoughts on the subject being discussed.

However, it became clear in our first session that Oz was not responding for any great length of time to this approach and thus we referred the group as a whole to the 'code of conduct' displayed on the wall. As a confident member from the start, Oz had been instrumental in producing these rules and thus we could use his own thoughts. This kind of indirect challenging of Oz's behaviour addressed to the group as a whole allowed us to re-direct his contributions ... Once the correct balance had been struck between participating and monopolising, Oz proved to be a valuable member of the group. Moreover, by providing us with the need to address an issue breaching group rules, Oz's behaviour aided the establishment of the group, as members recognised that any problems would be addressed fairly and that items such as the code of conduct were there to help the group.

Portfolio O, 5.2

BIBLIOGRAPHY

AASWG (1999) *Standards for Social Work Practice with Groups*, Association for the Advancement of Social Work with Groups: www.aaswg.org

Adams, J. (2004) 'Participant-focused questionnaires', *Groupwork*, 14.3, pp. 11–17, London: Whiting and Birch.

Argyle, E. and Bolton, G. (2004) 'The use of art within a groupwork setting', *Groupwork*, 14.1, pp. 46–62, London: Whiting and Birch.

Asch, S.E. (1952) *Social Psychology*, Englewood Cliffs, NJ: Prentice Hall.

Baggini, J. (2004) *What's It All About?*, London: Granta.

Barlow, J. (1997) *Systematic Review of the Effectiveness of Parent-training Programmes in Improving Behaviour Problems in Children Aged 3–10 Years*, Oxford: Health Services Research Unit, University of Oxford.

Belbin, R.M. (1993) *Team Roles at Work*, Oxford: Butterworth-Heinemann.

Berne, E. (1967) *Games People Play*, London: Penguin

Bertcher, H.J. (1994) *Group Participation: Techniques for Leaders and Members* (2nd edition), London: Sage.

Birnbaum, M. and Wayne, J. (2000) 'Group work content in foundation generalist education: the necessity for change', *Journal of Social Work Education*, 36, pp. 347–56.

Brower, A.M., Arndt, R.G. and Ketterhagen, A. (2004) 'Very good solutions really do exist for group work research design problems' in C.D. Garvin, L.M. Gutiérrez and M.J. Galinsky (eds) *Handbook of Social Work with Groups*, pp. 435–46, New York: Guilford Press.

Brown, A. (1994) *Groupwork* (3rd edition), Aldershot: Arena.

Carr, A. (2000) 'Evidence-based practice in family therapy and systemic consultation', *Journal of Family Therapy*, 22.1, pp. 29–60.

Cohen, M.B. and Mullender, A. (eds) (2003) *Gender and Groupwork*, London and New York: Routledge.

Constable, R. and Frysztacki, K. (1994) 'The context for practice and education in Polish social work: foundations for the international consultation process', in R. Constable and V. Mehta (eds) *Education for Social Work in Eastern Europe: Changing Horizons*, Chicago: Lyceum Books.

Coyle, G. (1937) *Studies in Group Behaviour*, New York and London: Harper and Brothers.

Croft, S. and Beresford, P. (2002) 'Service users "perspective" ', in Davies, M. (ed.) *The Blackwell Companion to Social Work*, pp. 385–93, Oxford: Blackwell Publishers.

Dixon, L. (2000) 'Punishment and the question of ownership: groupwork in the criminal justice system', *Groupwork*, 12.1, pp. 6–25, London: Whiting and Birch.

Doel, M. (2004) 'Difficult behaviour in groups', *Groupwork*, 14.1, pp. 80–100, London: Whiting and Birch.

Doel, M. and Sawdon, C. (1995) 'A strategy for groupwork education and training in a social work agency', *Groupwork*, 8.2, pp. 189–204, London: Whiting and Birch.

Doel, M. and Sawdon, C. (1999a) *The Essential Groupworker: Teaching and Learning Creative Groupwork*, London: Jessica Kingsley.

Doel, M. and Sawdon, C. (1999b) 'No group is an island: groupwork in a social work agency', *Groupwork*, 11.3, pp. 50–69, London: Whiting and Birch.

Doel, M. and Shardlow, S.M. (1995) *Preparing Post Qualifying Portfolios: A Practical Guide for Candidates*, London: Central Council for Education and Training in Social Work.

Doel, M., Sawdon, C. and Morrison, D. (2002) *Learning, Practice and Assessment: Signposting the Portfolio*, London: Jessica Kingsley.

Ebenstein, H. (1999) 'Single session groups: issues for social workers', in *Social Work with Groups*, 21.1/2, pp. 49–60.

Eraut, M. (2005) 'Continuity of learning', *Learning in Health and Social Care*, 4.1, pp. 1–6, Blackwell Science.

Fairbairn, G.J. (2002) 'Ethics, empathy and story-telling in professional development', *Learning in Health and Social Care*, 1.1, pp. 22–32, Blackwell Science.

Fatout, M.F. (1998) 'Exploring worker responses to critical incidents', *Groupwork*, 10.3, pp. 183–95, London: Whiting and Birch.

Forte, J.A. (1994) 'Around the world with social group work: knowledge and research contributions', *Social Work with Groups*, 17.2, pp. 143–62.

Fuchs, B. (2002) *Group Games: Social Skills*, Bicester: Speechmark.

Gant, L.M. (2004) 'Evaluation of group work', in C.D. Garvin, L.M. Gutiérrez, and M.J. Galinsky (eds) *Handbook of Social Work with Groups*, pp. 461–75, New York: Guilford Press.

Garvin, C.D., Gutiérrez, L.M. and Galinsky, M.J. (eds) (2004) *Handbook of Social Work with Groups*, New York: Guilford Press.

Gilbert, C. (2004) 'Documentation matters', unpublished paper: 26th annual conference of AASWG (Association for the Advancement of Social Work with Groups) Oct 2004, Detroit.

Gitterman, A. (2004) 'The mutual aid model', in C.D. Garvin, L.M. Gutiérrez, and M.J. Galinsky (eds) *Handbook of Social Work with Groups*, pp. 93–110, New York: Guilford Press.

Goleman, D. (1996) *Emotional Intelligence*, London: Bloomsbury.

Gould, B. and Masters, H. (2004) 'Learning to make sense: the use of critical incident analysis in facilitated reflective groups of mental health student nurses', *Learning in Health and Social Care*, 3.2, pp. 53–63, Oxford: Blackwell Science.

Groupwork (2004) *Social Action Themed Issue*, 14.2, London: Whiting and Birch.

Harrower, J. (1993) 'Groupwork with Young Offenders' in Dwivedi, K. (ed.) *Groupwork with Children and Adolescents*, London: Jessica Kingsley.

Henchman, D. and Walton, S. (1993) 'Critical incident analysis and its application in groupwork', *Groupwork*, 6.3, pp. 189–198, London: Whiting and Birch.

Horwath, J. and Calder, M.C. (1998) 'Working together to protect children on the child protection register: myth or reality?', *Groupwork*, 13.1, pp. 57–72, London: Whiting and Birch.

Hutchings, S., Hall, J. and Loveday, B. (2003) *Teamwork*, Bicester: Speechmark.

Johnson, D.W. and Johnson, F.P. (1994) *Joining Together: Group Theory and Group Skills* (5th edition), Boston, MA: Allyn and Bacon.

Johnson, P., Beckerman, A. and Auerbach, C. (2001) 'Researching our own practice: single system design for groupwork', *Groupwork*, 13.1. pp. 57–72, London: Whiting and Birch.

Jordan, B. (2004) Emancipatory social work? Opportunity or oxymoron, *British Journal of Social Work*, 34, pp. 5–19.

Lähteenmäki, M.-L. (2005) 'Reflectivity in supervised practice', *Learning in Health and Social Care*, 4.1, pp. 18–28, Oxford: Blackwell Science.

Lee, F.W. and Yim, E.L. (2004) 'Experiential learning group for leadership development of young people', *Groupwork*, 14.3, pp. 63–90, London: Whiting and Birch.

Le Riche, P. and Tanner, K. (eds) (1998) *Observation and Its Application to Social Work – Rather Like Breathing*, London: Jessica Kingsley.

Lewis, J. (2002) 'The contribution of research findings to practice change', *MCC Building Knowledge for Integrated Care*, 10.1, pp. 9–12.

Lizzio, A. and Wilson, K. (2001a) 'Facilitating group beginnings – a practice model', *Groupwork*, 13.1, pp. 6–30, London: Whiting and Birch.

Lizzio, A. and Wilson, K. (2001b) 'Facilitating group beginnings – from basic to working engagement', *Groupwork*, 13.1, pp. 31–56, London: Whiting and Birch.

Magen, R. (2004 'Measurement issues', in C.D. Garvin, L.M. Gutiérrez and M.J. Galinsky (eds) *Handbook of Social Work with Groups*, pp. 447–60, New York: Guilford Press.

Malekoff, A. (1999) 'Expressing our anger: hindrance or help in groupwork with adolescents', *Groupwork*, 11.1, pp. 71–83, London: Whiting and Birch.

Manor, O. (2000a) *Choosing a Groupwork Approach: An Inclusive Stance*, London: Jessica Kingsley.

Manor, O. (ed.) (2000b) *Ripples: Groupwork in Different Settings*, London: Whiting and Birch.

Maram, M. and Rice, S. (2002) 'To share or not to share: dilemmas of facilitators who share the problem of group members', *Groupwork*, 13.2, pp. 6–33, London: Whiting and Birch.

Marsh, P. and Doel, M. (2005) *The Task-Centred Book*, London: Routledge/ Community Care.

Mayadas, N.S., Smith, R. and Elliott, D. (2004) 'Social group work in a global context', in C.D. Garvin, L.M. Gutiérrez and M.J. Galinsky (eds) *Handbook of Social Work with Groups*, pp. 45–57, New York: Guilford Press.

Mayo, M. (1997) 'Community Work', in R. Adams, L. Dominelli and M. Payne (eds) *Social Work: Themes, Issues and Critical Debates*, London: Macmillan.

McDermott, F. (2005) 'Researching groupwork: outsider and insider perspectives', *Groupwork*, 15.1, pp. 91–109, London: Whiting and Birch.

Meier, A. (2004) 'Technology-mediated groups', in C.D. Garvin, L.M. Gutiérrez and M.J. Galinsky (eds) *Handbook of Social Work with Groups*, pp. 479–505, New York: Guilford Press.

Mistry, T. and Brown, A. (eds) (1997) *Race and Groupwork*, London: Whiting and Birch.

Mullender, A. and Ward, D. (1991) *Self-Directed Groupwork: Users Take Action for Empowerment*, London: Whiting and Birch.

Northen, H. (2004) 'Ethics and values in group work', in C.D. Garvin, L.M. Gutiérrez and M.J. Galinsky (eds) *Handbook of Social Work with Groups*, pp. 76–89, New York: Guilford Press.

O'Connor, I. (1992) 'Bereaved by suicide: setting up an "ideal" therapy group in a real world', *Groupwork*, 5.3, pp. 74–86, London: Whiting and Birch.

Papell, C.P. and Rothman, B. (1968) 'Social group work models: possession and heritage', *Journal of Education for Social Work*, 2, pp. 66–77.

Parsloe, E. and Wray, M. (2000) *Coaching and Mentoring*, London: Kogan Page.

Pawson, R., Boaz, A., Grayson, L., Long, A. and Barnes, C. (2003) *Types and Quality of Knowledge in Social Care*, SCIE Knowledge Review 3, London: Social Care Institute for Excellence.

Peake, A. and Otway, O. (1990) 'Evaluating success in groupwork; why not measure the obvious?', *Groupwork*, 3.2, pp. 118–33, London: Whiting and Birch.

Phillips, J. (2001) *Groupwork in Social Care*, London: Jessica Kingsley.

Pitts, J. (1999) *Working With Young Offenders*, Basingstoke: Macmillan.

Pollio, D. (2002) 'The evidence-based group worker', *Social Work with Groups*, 25.4, pp. 57–70, Haworth Press.

Preston-Shoot, M. (2004) 'Evidence – the final frontier? Star Trek, groupwork and the mission of change', *Groupwork*, 14.3, pp. 18–43, London: Whiting and Birch.

Reid, K. (1988) ' "But I don't want to lead a group!" Some common problems of social workers leading groups', *Groupwork*, 1.2, pp. 124–34, London: Whiting and Birch.

Richmond, M. (1917) *Social Diagnosis*, New York: Russel Sage Foundation.

Rishty, A.C. (2000) 'The strengths perspective in reminiscence groupwork with depressed older adults', *Groupwork*, 12.3, pp. 37–55, London: Whiting and Birch.

Rooney, R. and Chovanec, M. (2004) 'Involuntary groups', in C.D. Garvin, L.M. Gutiérrez and M.J. Galinsky (eds) *Handbook of Social Work with Groups*, pp. 212–26, New York: Guilford Press.

Rose, S.D. (2004) 'Cognitive-behavioural group work', in C.D. Garvin, L.M. Gutiérrez and M.J. Galinsky (eds) *Handbook of Social Work with Groups*, pp. 111–35, New York: Guilford Press.

Rushton, A. and Martyn, H. (1990) 'Two post-qualifying courses in social work: the views of the course members and their employers', *British Journal of Social Work*, 20, pp. 445–68.

Schwartz, W. (1961) 'The social worker in the group', *New Perspectives on Services to Groups: Theory, Organisation, Practice*, New York: National Association of Social Workers.

Senge, P.M. (1990) *The Fifth Discipline: The Art and Practice of the Learning Organization*, New York: Doubleday.

Sharry, J. (1999) 'Building solutions in groupwork with parents', *Groupwork*, 11.2, pp. 68–89, London: Whiting and Birch.

Sharry, J. (2001) *Solution-Focused Groupwork*, London: Sage.

Sharry, J. and Fitzpatrick, C. (2001) *Parents Plus Facilitators Manual*, www.parentsplus.ie.

Shaw, I., Arskey, H. and Mullender, A. (2004) *How Knowledge Works in Social Care Report: ESRC Research, Social Work and Social Care*, London: Social Care Institute for Excellence.

Sheffield, A.E. (1920) *Social Case History*, New York: Russel Sage Foundation.

Sheldon, B. (2002) 'Cognitive behavioral methods in social care: a look at the evidence' in Stepney, P. and Ford, D. (eds) *Social Work Models, Methods and Theories: A Framework for Practice*, pp. 65–83, Lyme Regis: RHP.

Sheldon, B. and MacDonald, G. (forthcoming) *A Textbook of Social Work*, London:Routledge.

Sheppard, M., Newstead, S., DiCaccavo, A. and Ryan, K. (2001) 'Comparative hypothesis assessment and quasi-triangulation as process knowledge assessment strategies in social work practice', *British Journal of Social Work*, 31, pp. 863–85.

Shulman, L. (1999) *The Skills of Helping Individuals, Families, Groups and Communities* (4th edition), Itasca, IL: Peacock.

Silverlock, M. (2000) 'Learning beyond the classroom: a role for groupwork', *Groupwork*, 12.1, pp. 58–71, London: Whiting and Birch.

Simmond, M. (2005) 'Practicing to learn: occupational therapy with the children of Viet Nam', in F. Kronenberg, S. Simo Algado and N. Pollard (eds) *Occupational Therapy without Borders*, Elsevier.

Smale, G.D. (1996) *Mapping Change and Innovation*, London: HMSO.

Smokowski, P.R., Galinsky, M. and Harlow, K. (2001) 'Technology-based groups', *Groupwork*, 13.1, pp. 98–115, London: Whiting and Birch.

Springer, D.W., Pomeroy, E.C. and Johnson, T. (1999) 'A group intervention for children of incarcerated parents: initial blunders and subsequent solutions', *Groupwork*, 11.1, pp. 54–70, London: Whiting and Birch.

St Thomas, B. and Johnson, P. (2002) 'In their own voices: play activities and art with traumatised children', *Groupwork*, 13.2, pp. 34–48, London: Whiting and Birch.

Staples, L.H. (2004) 'Social action groups', in C.D. Garvin, L.M. Gutiérrez and M.J. Galinsky (eds) *Handbook of Social Work with Groups*, pp. 344–60, New York: Guilford Press.

The Thursday Girls (2004) *A Life to Live: A Group Journey with Advanced Breast Cancer*, Carlton, NA: PyschOz Publications.

Tolman, R.M. and Molidor, C.E. (1994) 'A decade of social group work research: trends in methodology, theory and program development', *Research on Social Work Practice*, 4.2, pp. 142–59.

TOPSS (2002) *National Occupational Standards for Social Work*, Training Organisation for Personal Social Services. www.topss.org.uk/uk eng/framesets/engindex.htm.

Trevithick, P. (2005) *Social Work Skills* (2nd edition), Buckingham: Open University Press.

Tuckman, B.W. (1965) 'Developmental sequences in small groups', *Psychological Bulletin*, 63, pp. 384–99.

Tuckman, B.W. and Jensen, M.A. (1977) 'Stages of small group development revisited', *Group and Organizational Studies*, 2, pp. 419–27.

Walker, D. (1985) 'Writing and reflection', in D. Boud, R. Keogh and D. Walker (eds) *Reflection: Turning Experience into Learning*, pp. 52–68, Worcester: Billing and Sons.

Ward, D. (2002) 'Groupwork', in R. Adams, L. Dominelli and M. Payne (eds) *Social Work: Themes, Issues and Critical Debates* (2nd edition), Basingstoke: Macmillan.

Ward, D. (2004) 'Editorial introducing Social Action theme issue', *Groupwork*, 14.2, London: Whiting and Birch.

Wayne, J. and Cohen, C.S. (2001) *Group Work Education in the Field*, Alexandria, VA: Council on Social Work Education.

Webster-Stratton, C. and Herbert, M. (1994) *Troubled Families, Problem Children*, Chichester: Wiley.

Wenger, E., McDermott, R. and Snyder, W.M. (2002) *Cultivating Communities of Practice*, Cambridge, MA: Harvard Business School Press.

Yates, J. (2004) 'Evidence, effectiveness and groupwork developments in youth justice', *Groupwork*, 14.3, pp. 112–32, London: Whiting and Birch.

INDEX